The
COMPLETE BOOK
of BREAST CARE

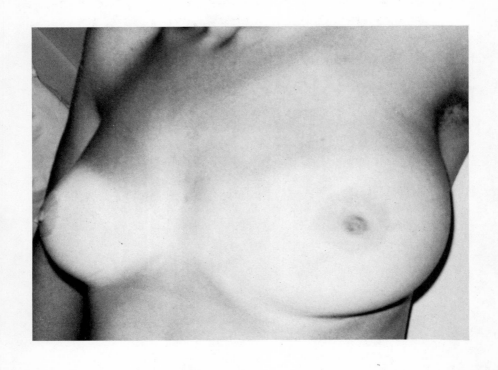

The
COMPLETE BOOK
of BREAST CARE

BY

ROBERT E. ROTHENBERG, M.D., F.A.C.S.

A Medbook Publication

CROWN PUBLISHERS, INC.
NEW YORK

Other Books Written or Edited by the Au

GROUP MEDICINE AND HEALTH INSURANC
UNDERSTANDING SURGERY
THE NEW ILLUSTRATED MEDICAL ENCYCLOPEDIA
FOR HOME USE
THE NEW AMERICAN MEDICAL DICTIONARY
and HEALTH MANUAL
HEALTH IN THE LATER YEARS
REOPERATIVE SURGERY
THE NEW ILLUSTRATED CHILD CARE ENCYCLOPEDIA
FOR THE HOME
THE DOCTORS' PREMARITAL MEDICAL ADVISER
THE FAST DIET BOOK
THE COMPLETE HOME MEDICAL ENCYCLOPEDIA &
GUIDE TO FAMILY HEALTH
THE COMPLETE SURGICAL GUIDE
WHAT EVERY PATIENT WANTS TO KNOW
THE FAMILY HEALTH & MEDICAL RECORD BOOK
(in press)

Library of Congress Cataloging in Publication Data

Rothenberg, Robert E.
The complete book of breast care.

"A Medbook publication."
Includes index.
1. Breast—Care and hygiene. 2. Breast—Diseases.
I. Title. [DNLM: 1. Breast—Popular Works.
2. Breast diseases—Popular works. 3. Breast neo-
plasms—Popular works. WP840 R846c]
RG493.R67   618.1'9   74-30108
ISBN 0-517-51909-7

Acknowledgments

In preparing this book I have relied heavily upon the knowledge of colleagues who specialize in one or another aspect of breast disorder. Adequate treatment of the breast requires a team effort, often employing the expertise of the radiologist, the pathologist, the epidemiologist, the chemotherapist, the geneticist, the plastic surgeon, the obstetrician, the gynecologist, the endocrinologist, and the breast surgeon. To them, I have turned frequently for information. In particular, I wish to thank Doctors Daniel Choy, Michel de Cordier, Edouardo Dazo, Roger Hassid, Leo Keller, Paul Metzger, Guy Robbins, Sidney Silverstone, Cyril Solomon, Philip Strax, and Joseph Tamerin for the time they so generously gave to this enterprise. Some contributed vital statistical data to support the main thesis of this work; others lent X-rays, line drawings, and photographs for reproduction; and still others spent long hours in discussing with me their particular points of view relative to the origin, diagnosis, and treatment of various breast problems. My special thanks go to the forty professors of surgery at medical colleges throughout the country who took the trouble to answer a questionnaire relating to certain controversial aspects of the treatment for diseases of the breast.

To the American Cancer Society, the Reach for Recovery Program, the Label Division of the International Ladies Garment Workers Union, and to the Metropolitan Life Insurance Company, I wish to express gratitude for permission to reprint pertinent data and diagrams.

Lastly, I wish to thank my good friend and assistant Roberta Hatch for her great cooperation in collating material and getting the manuscript into shape for publication.

Illustrations not from the author's collection are by the courtesy of Abradale Press (*The Complete Home Medical Encyclopedia and Guide to Family Health*): pages 2, 5, 38, 105, 125, 129, 138, 158, 169; Dell Publishing Co., Inc. (*The New Illustrated Child Care Encyclopedia for the Home*): page 22; Michael F. De Cordier, M.D.: pages 131, 140, 227; W. B. Saunders Co. (*Diseases of the Breast*): page 148; Memorial Sloan-Kettering Cancer Center and the American Cancer Society: pages 209–14.

R. E. R.

CONTENTS

Preface

It is remarkable that the breasts, so superficially located, so easily examined, and so often touched and handled by the woman and her mate, can harbor so many disorders that go undetected for months or years at a time. If one could encourage more women to be as *medically* breast-conscious as they are *aesthetically* breast-conscious, much unnecessary suffering could be averted.

This book deals with the healthy breast as well as the diseased breast. It concentrates on the adult female breast but also considers conditions affecting the breast during childhood, adolescence, and in the later years; it even includes the male breast. Within these pages are discussions of breast anatomy and function, the breast as a sex organ and as a symbol of pride and beauty (or the source of shame and unhappiness), even plastic surgery of the breast. However, the major aim of this work is to help save lives by pointing out ways to combat breast disease through early detection and intelligent selection of the best course of treatment.

Medical statistics show that one of four women in the United States develops some type of breast disorder, from minor to major significance, requiring treatment. And if the current incidence continues without substantial change over the next few decades, approximately one out of fourteen women at some time in her life is destined to get breast cancer. The enormity of this problem can be appreciated when one considers the latest United States Census figures of 70 million females eighteen years of age and older. The extremely high incidence of breast disease may be attributed in no small measure to the fact that the mammary glands in their structure and function are subjected to repeated fluctuations by the various cycles through which women pass. The breasts, if one can personify them, are confused each month when they get ready for a pregnancy that doesn't take place; then, when a pregnancy eventually does occur, the breasts respond by undergoing major structural and physiological changes in their blood circulation and in the secretory function of their glands, only to discover after childbirth that the changes were all for naught when the mother decides not to nurse her child. Thus the sole purpose for which the breasts were created is vitiated. Later on, when menopause approaches and the breasts get ready to settle down to a life of inactivity, they are often called upon to act like youngsters when their host takes large doses of female sex hormones.

Another reason for the extraordinary number of disorders is that the breast is a satellite organ, dependent on the activities of distant controlling hormones produced by the pituitary gland in the base of the brain, the adrenal glands above the kidneys, and most important, the ovaries. Upsets in the normal functioning of these glands and disturbance in their interaction with one another frequently cause breast disorder. Also, one must consider that the breast matures very late, and is called upon to do so at an extremely rapid rate during the few intensely stressful years of adolescence, unlike the leisurely development of other organs that proceed in the quiet, comfortable confines of a mother's womb. Lastly, the breasts are in an exposed position where they are unprotected and thereby subject to direct injury.

Within the past few years great attention has focused on differing views relating to the treatment of certain breast diseases and on the right of the patient to choose the form of therapy for a particular disorder. Discussion on this subject is aired frequently on popular television shows and is written about often in magazines and the daily press. Arguments are being advanced by so-called breast authorities—who should really know better—that it matters relatively little what specific kind of treatment a patient receives for breast cancer: the outcome will be more or less the same. It is one of the objectives of this book to show that this contention is far from the truth.

By a curious misconstruction of the meaning of women's rights, it has been propounded by some of the lay public, and supported by a few confused people in the medical profession, that the patient rather than the doctor should make the final decision as to what operation is to be performed for a particular breast condition. Along with the great majority of surgeons in this country, I believe fully in the recently enunciated Patient's Bill of Rights. This means that the patient has a right to know all the facts concerning his or her illness and the proposed treatment. It gives the patient the right to reject any type of treatment after all the facts have been presented. It does not mean, however, that the surgeon should abandon his vitally important role in persuading the patient to select the form of therapy he knows will afford the greatest chances for cure. Relative to this issue, the erudite physician in charge of medical affairs for the American Cancer Society writes:

> Surgeons advising mastectomy have occasionally been depicted as the "enemy" or sadomasochistic male chauvinists who seemingly enjoy excising the female breast while giving no thought to the psychological impact of mastectomy. A nationwide series of television "debates" between the proponents of conservatism and the traditionalist "radical" surgeons seem preplanned to generate controversy rather than to inform the public about the need for earlier diagnosis of breast cancer. One television producer recently rejected the appearance of a noted surgeon because his views were not sufficiently controversial to attract a large viewing audience.*

When we consider the huge number of women who will some day develop breast disease, we must feel keenly the need to set the record straight. There should be no place for physicians with meager statistics based on too limited an experience in the field of breast disease to pontificate on television, in books, in popular magazines, in such a manner as to cause confusion where no confusion is necessary. Their advice, expressed dogmatically to huge audiences who are poorly equipped to make their own judgment, may cost thousands of lives.

And we can't even consider surgery to be the only treatment, the ideal treatment, or the final answer to the cure of all breast disease. It does

* Arthur I. Holleb, M.D., writing in the magazine *Ca,* May/June, 1973.

represent, however, the best method presently available for treating most breast tumors. But many breast conditions will subside spontaneously, requiring no therapy, and other disorders may respond to hormone therapy or chemotherapy, or to irradiation. We will discuss all these matters.

But as I shall demonstrate later in this book, in the final analysis, it is up to each woman to help herself. She should practice monthly self-examination and undergo semiannual checkups by a physician who is an expert in the field of breast disease. If an abnormal condition is found, she should follow the expert's advice and shun medical faddists and those who lean toward sensationalism rather than adhering to documented facts. Then and only then would women be taking meaningful steps in the fight to reduce the numbers who die needlessly from malignant breast disease.

1 THE SIZE, SHAPE, AND ANATOMY OF THE BREAST

The term *mammal* is used to designate that group of animals with milk-secreting glands, or breasts. Most mammals are endowed by nature with a sufficient number of breasts to adequately nurse their young. Thus, animals with large litters may have four, five, or more pairs of breasts, whereas mammals, such as man and monkey, have a single pair.

The human breasts are located in the superficial tissues of the chest wall. In the adult female, the glands usually extend from the second or third to the fifth or sixth rib. Underlying the breasts are the pectoral muscles, which extend from the chest wall to the shoulder and to the collarbone. Through the center of the nipple is one larger and several smaller openings of the milk (lactiferous) ducts, which arise from the deeper tissues and connect with the glandular structures responsible for milk production. Surrounding the central portion of the nipple is a colored, circular area of skin known as the *areola,* from one to three inches in diameter. The size tends to be an inherited characteristic. The areola normally varies in color from a light pink to a dark brown, depending on the general complexion of the individual. During pregnancy, it often darkens in color and may remain that way after childbirth.

The breast is made up of approximately twenty *lobes,* each lobe emptying into its own milk duct, which terminates in the nipple. Just

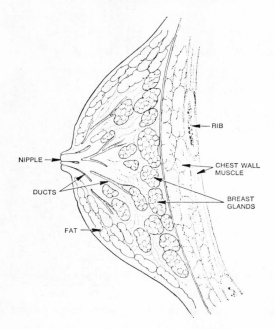

Anatomy of the female breast.

beneath the surface of the nipple these milk ducts coalesce to form a large cone-shaped area from which most of the milk will be extruded. The lobes are divided into a huge number of *lobules,* each containing approximately one hundred or more small glands that are grouped around a collecting milk duct. In addition to the glandular tissue within the breast, there is a lesser or greater amount of fat, nerves, arteries, veins, and lymphatic channels, which carry lymph to the lymph glands. There are also connective tissue fibers that mingle with the gland structure and help shape the organ into its rounded, conical form.

The size of the breast is determined both by the amount of gland tissue and the amount of fat it contains. Women with large, well-developed breasts usually have more gland tissue as well as more fat—generally, the stouter the female, the larger her breasts, and vice versa. The rounded form of the breast is most prominent in late adolescence and early adulthood, with a normal tendency for the breast to flatten out and sag after several offspring have been born and as menopause approaches. The loss

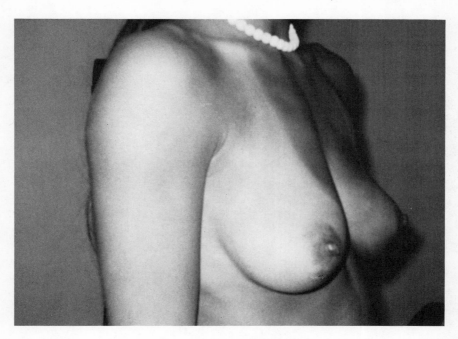

Breasts in young women who have not yet borne children tend to be round and firm, with nipples pointing straight out.

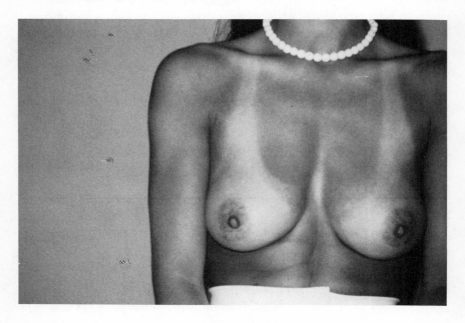

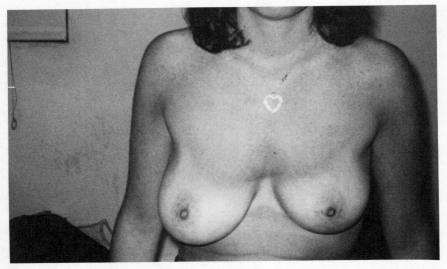

Dissimilar-sized breasts often cause young women to develop a sense of shame. As a result they try to hide their breasts.

of the conical, upright, rounded appearance of the breast is caused more often by a decrease in the amount of fat than to actual loss of gland tissue. Sagging may also be caused by a laxity and weakening of the fibrous connective tissue within the breast.

In the great majority of females, one breast is slightly larger than the other. Also, some females are naturally high-breasted whereas others are low-breasted. In the former, the upper part of the breast arises at the level of the second rib whereas in the latter group, the upper portion of the breast arises from the level of the third rib or the space between the third and fourth ribs. Some women have a nipple located directly in the middle of the breast whereas in others, the nipple occupies a lower position, thus giving the appearance of a sagging breast.

The nipple contains small muscle fibers that enable it to contract and become erect, or to relax and flatten out. Erection of the nipples takes place during suckling, during exposure to cold, or upon manipulation. The nipple is composed of erogenous tissue, similar to that of the tip of the penis. The skin of the nipple has no hair but does have a large number of sebaceous glands secreting an oily substance known as sebum. These glands surround the openings of the milk ducts. Some of these glands

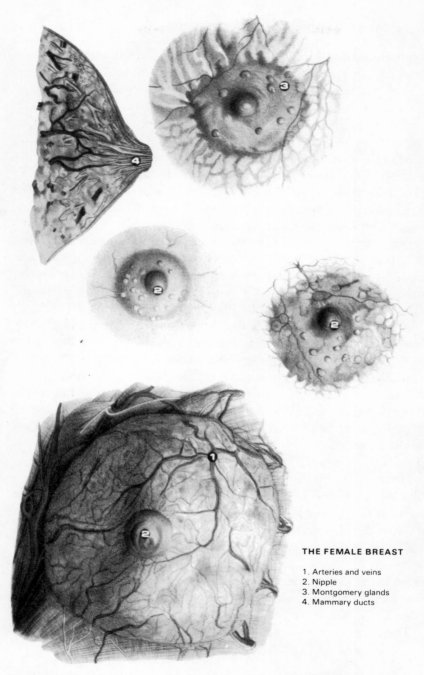

THE FEMALE BREAST

1. Arteries and veins
2. Nipple
3. Montgomery glands
4. Mammary ducts

The breasts are composed of nipples, milk ducts, glandular tissues, and surrounding fat and blood vessels.

are quite prominent, occasionally causing a woman to think that she has an abnormal structure within her nipple. These structures, known as Montgomery glands, tend to enlarge during pregnancy. Around the areola some women have a considerable number of well-developed follicles from which hair grows. Others have poorly developed follicles from which no hair grows.

At birth, some newborns have swollen breasts that discharge milk for a few days. This occurs in males as well as females and is thought to be caused by stimulation of the breasts by hormones circulating in the mother's blood. The hormone is transmitted from the mother to the unborn infant through the placenta. After childbirth, there is sufficient hormone left over in the newborn's blood to cause the breast to secrete milk. As days pass, this hormone disappears from the infant's bloodstream, and the breast stops secreting and returns to normal size. In rare instances, infection develops in a newborn's swollen breast and an abscess forms. In this event, surgical incision and drainage must be carried out.

Although the female tends to inherit the size, shape, and type of her breast, it is possible that she may inherit the type of breast that comes through the genes of her father rather than her mother. When this happens, the daughter's breast may not resemble her mother's breast at all. By the same token, the age at which the breast matures may follow the mother's or father's pattern of maturity. If a child has inherited genes of early development from her father's side of the family, she may develop breasts at an early age even though her mother's breasts may have developed during late puberty.

However, the breast normally begins to show signs of maturing when a child reaches ten to twelve years of age. Thus, the breast is the first organ to herald the onset of puberty. Breast enlargement is seen even before hair develops under the arms or in the pubic area, and may occur several years before the onset of menstruation.

Among Caucasians, particularly those who live in the more temperate climates, breast development tends to take place a year or two later than among people who live in tropical areas or among Orientals and blacks. The reason for this is not known.

There can be a wide age range in breast development. Some girls ten years of age have rather fully developed breasts whereas other children, normal in every respect, do not show breast growth until the fourteenth or fifteenth year of life. Since all normal children eventually do mature, late development should not cause concern. Certainly, hormone therapy should not be undertaken merely because an otherwise normal child happens to be a late bloomer.

Although the breast is subject to a considerable number of congenital and development abnormalities, the incidence is less than that of most other organs. Among the anomalies of the breast is *amastia,* the absence of a breast, which we will go into more thoroughly later. We will also refer to axillary breasts. In some women, there is an abnormal extension of breast tissue into the armpit, or axillary, region. Normally, there is a small amount of breast tissue extending up toward the armpit but it is considered abnormal when such tissue is located within the armpit, far from the chest wall, and grows to unusual proportions.

There are also supernumerary or accessory nipples, which occur as often in males as in females. We will go into this more thoroughly in the chapter on nipples, and also include a discussion on inverted nipples, which interferes with nursing and sexual stimulation. Dissimilar breasts should be mentioned also. Although the size of a woman's breasts are seldom exactly the same, it is considered abnormal when one breast is much larger than the other. Occasionally, the disparity is so great that a woman will wish to undergo plastic surgery to equalize them.

There is also hypertrophy of the breast. This is a condition in which one or both breasts become tremendously overgrown during puberty or pregnancy. When it takes place during puberty, it is usually not associated with abnormal gland function elsewhere in the body. The cause of hypertrophy during pregnancy is thought to be associated with increased hormone secretion and stimulation.

In certain cases, the overgrowth of the breast approaches four, five, or more times normal. Unfortunately, such a breast retains its huge size even beyond adolescence, and even after pregnancy has been concluded. People with breast hypertrophy suffer greatly both physically and psychologically. Fortunately, the condition can be corrected through plastic surgery.

Questions and Answers

By what age do breasts attain their full size?
Usually, by the seventeenth year in Caucasians; a year or two earlier in black and some Oriental races.

Can one make the nipples firmer?
Daily massaging of the nipples formerly was advocated during the early days of pregnancy in order to "firm them up" for eventual nursing. However, unless the nipples are inverted, this practice is no longer advised.

What is the blood supply to the breast?
Its main supply is derived from the internal mammary artery.

How many lymph glands (nodes) drain the breast area?
Approximately 30 to 40.

Where are the lymph glands located?
The armpit (axilla); above the collarbone (the supraclavicular region); and beneath the breastbone (the internal mammary area).

Can one strengthen the muscles of the breast?
The breast has no muscles although there are muscles—the pectoralis, major and minor—on the chest wall immediately beneath the breast. When these muscles are strong, their contraction may cause some motion of the overlying breast. However, true strengthening of the breast doesn't take place no matter how well developed the pectoral muscles are.

Do extra nipples ever enlarge during adolescence?
Occasionally, if there is gland tissue underlying the nipple. This occurs infrequently.

What can be done to alter the size of the nipples?
They cannot be made larger, but through plastic surgery, it is possible to make them smaller. However, this procedure is not often requested or performed.

Can the size of the mature breast be predicted during childhood?

No. The size of a child's nipple is no indication as to the eventual size of the mature breast.

Are the breasts ever larger during the later adolescent years than when a woman is fully matured?

Yes. Breasts are usually at their fullest during the period between 17 and 22 years of age.

Is enlargement of the breasts ever seen in little girls?

Yes. This is an unusual condition, but occasionally it is seen in children during their first three years of life. In some instances, there may be enlargement of one breast only. Such enlargement may indicate the presence of a tumor in the ovary, the adrenal gland, or the pineal gland within the brain.

What happens to abnormally large breasts in a child?

Sometimes, they subside spontaneously; in other instances, they continue to grow along with other evidences of precocious puberty. Such precocity may or may not be associated with a tumor in other organs.

Are exceptionally large breasts in a child under ten years of age ever an indication that she is suffering from a tumor in an ovary, adrenal gland, or pineal gland?

In some cases only. However, thorough investigation is indicated in all such children to rule out the presence of a tumor.

Is lack of breast development usually a sign of hormone deficiency?

Usually not. Most females with small breasts have normally developed organs of reproduction.

Is a woman with very small breasts less likely to be interested in sex than one with large well-developed breasts?

No. Breast size has nothing to do with sex interest or appetite.

Will repeated intercourse cause the breasts to enlarge?

No.

What effect can brassieres have on breast size?

None. They merely make the breasts appear smaller or larger.

Will the wearing of an uplift brassiere cause the breast to become less pendulous?

No, but it will appear less so.

How effective is cosmetic surgery in enlarging a breast?

Breast augmentation is a very successful operation to make the breast *appear* larger. See chapter 23.

2 BREAST FUNCTION

Originally, before the advent of bottle feeding, the breast was considered an essential part of the reproductive system. An offspring could not survive unless the mother nursed her child or, if she was lucky, found someone to act as a substitute or wet nurse. Today, in developed countries, with the use of cow's milk and milk substitutes, the breast has been relegated to a nonessential role in the reproductive cycle. Following its lessening of importance in the biological scheme of things, the breast developed a kind of aesthetic idealization. It became more an object of beauty and a structure whose use was devoted more to sexual gratification than to the feeding of the young. In this connection, one notes that in less well developed areas such as Africa, Asia, and parts of the Orient, where nursing is the rule rather than the exception, the breast is not often looked upon as an essential element of feminine pulchritude.

At birth, the breast has very little gland tissue. However, there are some functioning glands, as we have seen by the fact that the infant may secrete small quantities of milk within the first few days of life. When this episode ends, the breast enters a decade of inactivity. Then, between ten and twelve years of age, the nipple enlarges, becomes darker in color, and breast tissue forms beneath it. Glands, capable of eventually secreting milk, bud off from the milk ducts to increase the amount of total breast tissue. Breast growth usually begins a year or two before menstruation.

For several days prior to a menstrual period, the breast becomes larger, firmer, more nodular, and in many women, tender to the touch. These changes are preparatory to the possible onset of pregnancy. The added fullness of the premenstrual breast is thought to be due to increased blood supply and the retention of fluids caused by increased hormonal secretions by the ovaries. When pregnancy does not take place, the breasts subside and return to their normal state by the third or fourth day of menstruation.

When breasts become full prior to menstruation, it is more difficult for a surgeon to make an accurate determination of the presence or absence of a small lump. For this reason, surgeons often prefer to examine breasts at various times during the menstrual cycle. A true lump, not to be confused with the swelling that will accompany menstrual engorgement, will persist at all times during the month. A differential diagnosis between a lump requiring biopsy and one that can be left alone is not always easy. A condition known as cystic disease (covered in chapter 26), thought to be due to hormonal imbalance, can cause both breasts to feel lumpy throughout. This condition, too, should not be confused with the nodular feel to the normal breast that takes place prior to menstruation.

Girls between ten and fifteen years of age may not demonstrate normal breast growth if they suffer a lack of sufficient pituitary, thyroid, adrenal, or ovarian hormones. Delayed or even absent puberty is seen when these glands fail to function and are the seat of major maldevelopment or disease. Pituitary dwarfs may never have mature breasts; cretins who lack thyroid hormone have immature breasts, and pseudohermaphrodites with absence of functional ovaries will show no breast maturity. A severe nutritional deficiency can also delay breast development. I had a patient who had spent her twelfth to seventeenth years in a Nazi concentration camp during which time she was subject to continual starvation. She never menstruated or showed the slightest signs of breast growth until her release. On resuming an adequate diet, puberty rapidly ensued.

Within the first and second months of pregnancy, changes can be noted in the breast. It increases in size, feels firmer, and the nipple becomes larger and its color darkens slightly. These changes persist throughout the pregnancy. In the last few months of pregnancy the glands of the breast ready themselves for the secretion of milk. Immediately after the birth of the child a substance known as *colostrum* can be expressed from the nipple or is sucked from the breast by the nursing infant. Colostrum, composed of the debris that has been collecting within the glands and ducts of the breast during the last weeks of pregnancy, is thought to contain important antibodies beneficial to the newborn child. However, infants who fail to nurse do not seem to suffer from the lack of this substance.

If the infant nurses from the day of birth, the breast will begin to secrete milk in a day or two and will continue to do so as long as nursing takes place regularly. In certain isolated Eskimo tribes, mothers continued to nurse their children successfully for fifteen or sixteen years, until the offspring themselves got married.

When a mother decides not to nurse, a hormone known as Deladumone is injected soon after delivery, or stilbestrol is given by mouth for a few days to dry up the breasts. This usually works satisfactorily. If it is not used, caking of the breast may take place. This is a condition in which the milk becomes stagnant within the glands and ducts, causing considerable pain, swelling, and tenderness of the breast. If a mother nurses for several months and weans her baby slowly, caking seldom ensues and the breast dries up by itself within a week or two after nursing stops. In unusual instances, the breast continues to secrete milk indefinitely. This condition is thought to be caused by hormone imbalance. In rare cases, the breast fails to dry up because it is stimulated during the postpartum period. I encountered a patient who continued to secrete milk for five years after her last child was born. On questioning, it was revealed that her husband suckled her breasts regularly after she had stopped nursing. This practice never permitted a sufficient time for the breasts to dry up by themselves.

From the time childbearing ends until the onset of menopause, the breast is subject to the recurrent changes evoked by menstruation. This is approximately a twenty- to twenty-five-year span, during which the breast is called upon two hundred and fifty to three hundred times to react to the effects of changing quantities of ovarian hormones that circulate in the bloodstream. During these many years the human breast behaves unnaturally. If it were the breast of an animal, it would perform as nature intended it to, and would be involved each year with the host's pregnancy and would be nursed at regular intervals. Again, it is small wonder that the human breast is the seat of so many disorders.

As menopause approaches, the breast undergoes involution, and many of its functioning glands are replaced by fibrous tissue. There is a concomitant loss of fat tissue and a weakening of the connective tissue that binds all the tissues of the breast together. As a consequence of these changes, the breast flattens out, sags, becomes flabby, and its skin may wrinkle.

Questions and Answers

Do the breasts continue to mature prior to the onset of menstruation?
Yes. In some girls the breasts may be almost fully developed before menstruation begins.

Does the giving of hormones decrease the tenderness and engorgement of the breast prior to menstruation?
Not in most instances. Actually, it is poor practice to give hormones to treat this condition as they may aggravate it. Some doctors have urged the giving of male sex hormones in order to decrease breast engorgement but this, too, is not good practice.

Other physicians have administered diuretic medications to rid the body of excess fluids prior to the period. Most physicians feel that this is unwise practice as it may upset the chemical metabolism of the body.

Both of these forms of treatment may be likened to taking a sledgehammer to kill a fly.

Is there anything a woman can do to adjust to the tenderness and sensitivity of the breasts just prior to menstruation?
She might limit her fluid intake, and she may take an analgesic pill such as aspirin.

Does the weight of a woman influence breast function?
Not if her endocrine glands are functioning normally.

Are women with abnormal endocrine function more likely to develop breast cysts or tumors?
In all probability, yes. However, this is especially true for cysts and benign tumors. No proof exists that those with hormone imbalance are more prone to breast cancer.

Will abnormalities in function of the endocrine glands often influence a woman's ability to nurse a child?
If a woman has been able to give birth to a child, her endocrine glands function sufficiently well to permit nursing.

Does the breast of a virgin feel different from that of a nonvirgin?
No. Intercourse does not alter the appearance or the feel of a breast.

Does the breast of a woman who has borne children have a different feel from that of one who has not had a child?
Yes, to a slight degree. The breast of a woman who has had one or more children tends to feel somewhat softer and lies a bit flatter on the chest wall. These changes may be minimal or absent in some women.

At what stage of pregnancy do the breasts start to secrete?
Sometimes, during the last two or three months of pregnancy, a small amount of clear, yellow secretion appears from the nipples.

How soon after childbirth will the milk come in?
Within 24 to 48 hours if the breast is suckled; within 72 to 96 hours if the mother does not nurse.

Can all women nurse if they want to?
Yes, if their nipples are normal. However, not all women produce sufficient milk to satisfy the newborn. In rare instances, the infant rejects its mother's milk.

Is a woman who has never given birth to a child more likely to develop an upset in breast function?
It is *thought* so, but no accurate scientific data are available on this subject.

Is it essential that a woman nurse a child in order to maintain normal functioning of the breast?
No. Many who have never nursed retain normal breast function throughout life.

Does suckling of the breasts produce nerve reactions in other parts of the body?
Yes. It has been found that suckling causes nerve impulses to go to the brain and to stimulate the pituitary gland to secrete a hormone known

as oxytocin. This hormone is carried to the breast where it stimulates the glands to secrete milk into the duct system.

Also, suckling by a mate produces nerve reactions whereby the mucus glands in the vaginal region secrete and ready the individual for intercourse.

Will breast-feeding help the uterus to contract and return to normal size after childbirth?
Yes, as it stimulates the secretion of the hormone oxytocin, originating in the pituitary gland.

Do women who have breast-fed their children have less chance of developing cystic disease within the breast?
No. The tendency toward this condition usually precedes the period during which the woman became pregnant.

Will nursing a child cure cystic disease of the breast?
No.

Is breast function influenced by a hysterectomy?
Not if one or both ovaries have been left in place.

Is breast function influenced by removal of the ovaries?
Yes. The breasts will then undergo the natural changes seen with menopause.

3 WEIGHT AND THE BREASTS

The breast is influenced greatly by weight. When a woman is markedly obese for a long period of time, the fibrous connective tissue strands that run through the breast and attach it to the chest wall are stretched and weakened. Since these strands of tissue are not elastic, even when the woman loses her excess weight, they remain stretched and the breast continues to sag on the chest wall. Thus, the beauty of the high-positioned, rounded contour of the breast is permanently lost.

In some women, the breast becomes unattractively prominent due to the deposition of large amounts of fat within its substance. On the other hand, many obese adolescent girls and young women lament the fact that their breasts are so small. Rarely is this the result of glandular inadequacy. In most instances, the undersize is apparent rather than real. The surrounding tissues on the chest wall are so padded with fat that they hide the breasts' true size and contour. When the young woman sheds excess poundage the breast emerges from hiding and assumes its normal appearance.

In markedly overweight women the skin, too, stretches to accommodate the increased size of the breast. As the obesity continues, the elastic fibers within the skin lose some of their ability to contract, and even after these women lose weight, the skin remains stretched, and unsightly streaks appear. These streaks seldom disappear, thus creating a permanent disfigurement. Patients should be advised that their best chance not to develop the streaks is to lose weight gradually. Rapid weight loss is more conducive to the development of these blemishes.

Underweight women tend to have flat, flabby breasts since much of the roundness and firmness of the normal organ is created by the padding of the glandular tissues with surrounding fat. When normal weight is regained, the breast usually returns to its original size, shape, and position on the chest wall. The fibrous connective tissue within the breast and the overlying skin, not having been stretched during the period of underweight, regains its normal supportive functions.

Questions and Answers

Does the obese breast function as well as the underweight or normal breast?

Yes. The deposit of excess fat within the breast does not seem to affect its function. A fat mother can nurse as well as a thin one.

Why do some women with large breasts have a marked amount of sagging while the large breasts of others seem to retain their high position on the chest wall?

As we know, breast contours and positions differ greatly from one female to another. Some women have strong fibrous connective tissue within their breasts that, despite marked obesity or size, is capable of maintaining the high position of the breast on the chest wall.

Can permanent sagging of an overweight breast be prevented by the wearing of a good uplift brassiere?

Yes, to a limited extent. If such a brassiere is worn continuously, it may prevent stretching of the supportive fibers of the breast.

Is there anything except the wearing of a good uplift brassiere that can prevent the large breasts of the obese from sagging?

No.

Do obese women always show an increase in the size of their breasts?

No. Extra fat is deposited capriciously beneath the skin of the body. Some people seem to collect excess fat mainly in their abdominal region;

others collect it most around the hips and buttocks. By the same token, the breasts enlarge greatly in some obese women whereas others will show relatively little increase in the size of their breasts even though they have become markedly overweight.

Do the nipples become larger when one is obese?
Yes, because the skin is stretched. Since the nipples contain a great deal of elastic tissue, they usually return to normal size after the woman loses excess weight.

Will massage make fat breasts smaller?
No, and it may even damage the breasts if it is too strenuous. Hemorrhage within the breast secondary to massage is not infrequent.

Is there any such thing as spot-reducing to make large breasts smaller?
No.

Why is it that some overweight women have small breasts while some very thin women have large breasts?
Breast size is an inherited characteristic; weight is not.

Is it wise for a markedly overweight woman to have her breasts made smaller through plastic surgery?
No. It is not always possible to determine how much of the oversize of a woman's breast is due to obesity and how much is due to excess breast tissue. Therefore, before undertaking plastic surgery, it is important for the patient to return to normal body weight.

Is it possible that some women may lose weight and still retain oversized breasts?
Yes, if their breasts contain an excess of gland tissue.

What can be done to get rid of the streaking of the skin of the breasts that results from weight loss?
Nothing. Excess skin may be excised by a plastic surgeon, but this will merely substitute surgical scars for the streaking.

Do streaks from weight loss tend to disappear by themselves?
To a limited extent over a period of years.

Is an obese breast more apt to develop a tumor than a thin breast?
The breast in obese women is more likely to develop lipomas (fatty tumors). It is not more prone to cancer or other lesions.

4 ENDOCRINE GLANDS, HORMONES, AND THE BREAST *

In chapter 2, attention was called to some of the influences of the various endocrine glands on the breast. Here, it would perhaps be informative to give a more detailed description of those glands, their hormones, and how they affect the breast.

Endocrine glands are structures that produce chemicals known as hormones. These hormones are secreted into the bloodstream through which they travel to other organs of the body where they exert specific reactions. If the organ so affected is also an endocrine gland, it may be stimulated to produce its own hormone that is, in turn, sent through the bloodstream to affect still another organ. As an example, the pituitary gland at the base of the brain secretes a hormone that goes to the ovaries and stimulates them to produce estrogen, the female sex hormone. We have seen that when this ovarian hormone is secreted it stimulates the breast to become engorged and, if no pregnancy ensues, it stimulates the uterus to menstruate. The system of actions and reactions as described above takes place with other endocrine glands and it is therefore not unexpected that these mechanisms frequently get out of order. Smooth interaction of the various endocrine responses is essential for normal functioning of all the organs that make up the reproductive system, including the breasts.

* Hormone therapy for breast cancer is discussed in chapter 28.

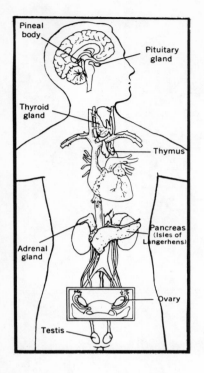

Endocrine glands, especially the pituitary, adrenals, and ovaries influence the breasts greatly.

One of the great difficulties in treating endocrine gland malfunction is the fact that few accurate tests are available to determine the amounts of hormones that are being secreted. There may be a lack or an excess of one or another hormone, but the diagnosis of this aberration cannot frequently be made by precise chemical determinations. More often than not, a diagnosis of pituitary, adrenal, or ovarian upset is made by observing the clinical symptoms, with a certain amount of educated guesswork thrown in.

Pituitary Gland

The pituitary gland, located beneath the brain, is called the master gland. Its hormones control the secretions of the other endocrine glands, namely, the thyroid gland, the parathyroid glands, the adrenal glands, the pancreas, the testicles, and the ovaries. If the pituitary gland fails to function properly during childhood, puberty may be delayed or not take place at all. The breasts, along with other organs of reproduction, may fail to mature. As pituitary failure is not a common condition, one rarely sees failure of breast development except when associated with dwarfism.

The main effect of the pituitary on the breast is through stimulation of the ovaries. Without adequate pituitary hormonal secretions the ovaries will not secrete the estrogen and progesterone that are considered essential for normal breast function. The breast, with disordered ovarian function, will not prepare itself for the cyclical changes it must undergo each month nor will it prepare itself properly for pregnancy and the ensuing childbirth. In addition, it is thought that several diseases of the breast originate because of ovarian dysfunction.

The pituitary gland is also thought to secrete a hormone known as prolactin, which stimulates the breast to secrete milk, and the hormone oxytocin, which causes the milk ducts to contract so that milk can be expelled from the breast.

Thyroid Gland

Although the thyroid gland is not directly involved in breast function or disease, its failure to function properly can have certain untoward effects. In cretinism little or no thyroid activity exists from birth. The child fails to grow and mature and, as a consequence, breast maturity fails to take place. Also, marked underactivity of the thyroid during otherwise normal adolescence is often associated with inadequate breast development. And inadequate thyroid secretion is sometimes accompanied by an inability of the woman to become pregnant and the breast cannot fulfill its true function.

The Ovaries

Apart from the pituitary, the breast is more dependent on the ovaries than on any other endocrine gland in the body. Within the monthly cycle its increase of estrogen causes the breast to become engorged and readies the body for pregnancy. When pregnancy occurs the ovaries secrete increased amounts of progesterone, which circulates in the body during pregnancy and readies the breast for ultimate lactation after childbirth. If pregnancy does not occur, estrogen secretion during that month will fall off and the breast will subside.

Cystic disease and intraductal papillomatosis are just two conditions, both benign, thought to originate in association with a marked imbalance in estrogen and progesterone secretions. Cystic disease of the breast exists to a greater or lesser degree in approximately 15 percent of all women between 35 and 50 years of age. The condition can be diagnosed readily by a characteristic lumpy feel throughout both breasts. (See chapter 26.) Intraductal papillomatosis is most often recognized by secretions that emanate from the nipple. (See chapter 24.)

Adrenal Glands

The breasts are also influenced by the amount of cortisone secreted by the adrenal glands. An excess of cortisone, caused either by abnormal gland function, a tumor in the adrenal, or by the taking of cortisone drugs for unrelated conditions, will result in a certain degree of suppression of estrogen production.

Some breast disorders are aggravated by the ill-advised taking of hormones without a physician's concurrence. For example, a woman with cystic disease should never take oral contraceptive medications unless she is under the care of a competent physician, gynecologist, or surgeon, as it may be instrumental in the formation of large cysts, or fluid-containing sacs. Estrogen should be prescribed cautiously to a woman with cystic disease—or intraductal papillomatosis—as it may stimulate the breast inordinately and exacerbate an existing condition. Considerable debate has surrounded the question whether oral contraceptives (which contain estrogen and progesterone) and estrogens can create disease within a normal breast. Most authorities don't believe so, but they agree that these can aggravate an existing condition.

Many patients who are given any form of hormone therapy want to know if a breast cancer can result from its use. On this question there is rather general agreement that cancer is not caused by hormone administration. On the other hand, some physicians do think that a dormant tumor might be activated and induced to grow with prolonged use of hormones.

One might assume that if an endocrine imbalance exists, it can be corrected by administration of the appropriate hormone. Thus, one might expect a breast disorder caused by a hormone imbalance to be readily overcome. Unfortunately, this is not true. Hormone therapy is notoriously unsuccessful in overcoming breast disorders and, in fact, the administration of hormones over a prolonged period of time may have harmful effects on the body mechanism, which far outweighs any possible benefit to the mammary gland. As an example, cystic disease of the breast usually persists throughout the entire childbearing period of a woman's life despite intensive hormone therapy and even repeated pregnancies and childbirths. But when menopause takes place and the ovarian secretions diminish, cystic disease of the breast subsides.

Questions and Answers

What effect does taking thyroid have on the breast?
None, if the breast is normally developed.

Can the use of face creams containing estrogen affect the breast?
Yes. In large quantities it will be associated with swelling and possible tenderness of the breast, along with increased sensitivity of the nipple.

Can ointments applied to the genital region affect the breast if they contain estrogen?
Yes, in the same manner as described above.

Does the placenta in a pregnant woman produce estrogen and progesterone, thus causing enlargement of the breasts?
Yes.

Is every doctor sufficiently knowledgeable to prescribe hormones for a breast disorder?
Hormones are rarely given to correct a breast disorder. Certainly, one should consult an endocrinologist or one who is very familiar with breast disorders before taking hormones therapeutically.

Should a woman on hormone treatment have her breasts examined regularly?
Yes, because the breast often reacts strongly to the taking of hormones.

Will the giving of hormones correct cystic disease of the breast?
Usually not.

Should a woman who has once had a cyst of the breast take hormones to prevent another one from forming?

Unfortunately, such treatment is not often effective.

If a woman has been taking hormones for a long period of time, is she more likely to develop a cancer of the breast?

No. There is no proof of this.

What is the effect of the male sex hormone upon the female breast?

1. Curiously, it may cause the breast to swell and become engorged.

2. When given to a woman who has just given birth to a child, it may dry up the milk.

3. When given to a woman with a breast cancer that has spread to other parts of the body, it may cause the cancer to regress for a period of time.

When one stops taking hormones does the breast usually return to its former state?

Yes.

5 BREAST DEVELOPMENT IN CHILDHOOD AND ADOLESCENCE

From a psychological point of view, it is very important that a girl know when to expect development of her breasts and how to react to it. Girls should be informed about the breasts as soon as they ask about them, usually when they have reached four to five years of age. Mothers should be open and frank in their discussions, and should not evade questions or make it seem "wrong" when the child evidences curiosity about the subject. Some mothers consciously hide their breasts from their daughters' view, thus creating the impression that the breast is something to be ashamed about.

Breast development becomes a problem when a girl is concerned because she is developing either faster or slower than her friends, or when she thinks her breasts are too small or too large. Because of these apprehensions, it is the mother's duty to reassure her daughter about normal variations in the timing of breast growth and in the variations in size. Frank discussions of these topics, when a girl is nine to ten years of age, will prevent unnecessary worry and embarrassment should she be either an early or late developer.

The breast in childhood is not subject to many diseases. Tumors of the breast in childhood are great rarities. Out of 70,000 deaths from breast cancer, only one was a child under ten years of age, and six were between the ages of fifteen and nineteen years. Among female adolescents benign tumors (fibroadenomas) of the breast are encountered, but it is not a frequent occurrence.

The most common breast abnormality of childhood, affecting both the male and female breast, is the so-called adolescent nodule. This is a smooth, rounded enlargement directly beneath the nipple, most usually seen in the tenth, eleventh, and twelfth years in girls and during the thirteenth, fourteenth, and fifteenth years in boys. The nodules first come to the attention of the children when they see the swelling, and concern mounts when the nipple develops tenderness to the touch. The cause for adolescent nodules is not precisely known but it is thought to result from the increased amount of hormones produced by the ovaries or testicles around the time of adolescence.

No medical or surgical treatment is necessary for the adolescent nodule. In most cases, it will disappear spontaneously within a few months. It becomes incorporated in developing breast tissue (one can distinguish between an adolescent nodule and normal breast growth by the fact that tenderness rarely accompanies the breast development of puberty).

A girl's breast should never be operated on and the nodule removed as the nodule may involve the entire breast tissue mass. If such a nodule is unwittingly removed, the girl may never develop a breast on that side.

Breast development not only takes place at varying ages, but each breast may develop at a different time. Unequal breast development often causes great concern but the child, and mother too, should be assured that the slow breast will eventually catch up to the fast one. There are exceptions, however, where one breast reaches full maturity while the other remains permanently underdeveloped. The reason for this is unknown, but it is considered to be a congenital defect about which nothing can be done during adolescence. When the girl reaches maturity, she may elect to have a plastic operation for *augmentation* of the underdeveloped breast.

Mothers often seek hormone therapy for their adolescent daughters who show late breast development. This form of treatment is contraindi-

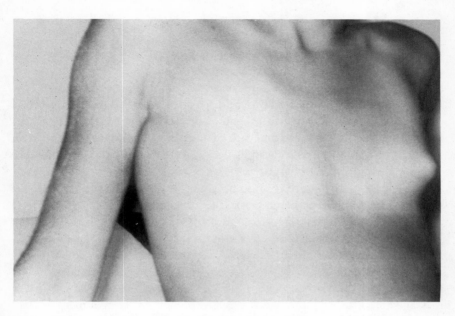

In prepuberty, the breasts may begin to develop at different times. This ten-year-old shows beginning development of the left breast only.

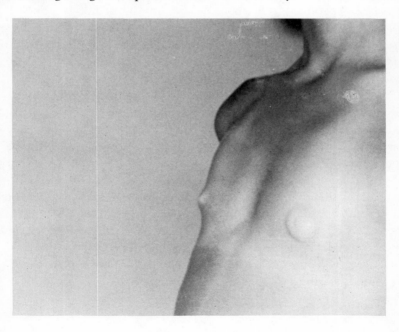

cated if the child's reproductive organs are normal. In other words, if a child's uterus and ovaries are anatomically normal and if she is menstruating normally, it is unwise to give hormones as they may upset glandular (endocrine) balance. However, if the child shows other signs of developmental abnormalities, such as absence of pubic and underarm hair, failure to develop female body contours, and lack of normal genital development, then hormone therapy may be indicated. For treatment, the parent should take the child to an endocrinologist who specializes in this type of disorder.

So great is the concern of some young women about the small size of their breasts that they become easy prey to commercial exploiters. There are many so-called "bust developers" on the market purporting to make breasts larger. It can be stated emphatically that these claims are false, and that there is nothing to be done to make breasts larger by the use of a mechanical device. Many so-called health experts advocate special exercises to enlarge the breasts but these, too, are ineffective. Others advise breast massage to "firm up" the breasts, but this method of treatment is also valueless. Finally, a word should be said about the use of hormone pills or ointments, and about the taking of oral contraceptives. Since the small breast is seldom caused by hormone deficiency or imbalance, it is unscientific to prescribe such medications to enlarge it. Though it is true that there may be some increase in the size of the breast if one takes estrogen pills or rubs in an estrogen ointment regularly, the dangers attendant on this course of action far outweigh the advantages of increased breast size. Ovarian and uterine function may be seriously disturbed by the ill-advised continued use of estrogens. Few women take oral contraceptives for the sole purpose of making their breasts look larger, but there is no doubt that in many instances breast swelling does occur. However, the increase in breast size is inconsequential.

Other adolescent girls are so disturbed about oversized breasts that they seek plastic surgery to reduce their size. In these cases, it is important to make a distinction between normally large breasts (a familial trait) and *hypertrophy* of the breasts, mentioned earlier, in which one or both breasts may be several times normal size. This condition should be treated by plastic surgery. To do otherwise would permit a young girl or woman to suffer unnecessarily.

Questions and Answers

Will a breast abscess in a newborn girl who secretes milk cause a deformity in the breast when she matures?

No. As the child grows older the scar of the incision to drain the abscess will become practically invisible.

Are children ever born without nipples?

The absence of nipples is an extremely rare congenital deformity. However, every once in a while a child is born with a normal nipple but with an absence of underlying breast tissue.

Does early breast development usually herald an early onset of menstruation?

Yes, the breasts, since they are an organ of sex, tend to develop about a year or two before menstruation starts.

Does premature breast development (between the ages of 8 and 10 years) usually signify an abnormal condition elsewhere in the body?

Not necessarily. There are many children who develop breasts precociously but are otherwise completely normal.

Are there tests that can tell whether a child with precocious breast development has some more serious generalized condition?

Yes, the pediatrician will probably test the function of the ovaries, the pituitary gland, and adrenal glands. These are the glands that must be investigated for tumor or disease if sexual development is precocious.

Is the size of a girl's breasts any indication of her ability to one day become pregnant?

If her organs of reproduction have developed normally and she is menstruating, breast size is of no consequence insofar as fertility is concerned.

Does a female ever reach full maturity with one breast developed and the other completely undeveloped?

Asymmetry of the breasts or late development of one breast is an unfortunate deformity about which little can be done. Perhaps when the child becomes an adult, she can consider one of the newer surgical procedures in which a plastic sac is inserted into the chest wall beneath the breast.

Should an adolescent girl with markedly enlarged breasts be operated upon to reduce their size?

Usually such a girl is overweight and if she returns to normal weight the breast enlargement decreases. However, if she has hypertrophy of the breasts, plastic surgery should be undertaken.

Should a parent permit an adolescent girl to pad her brassiere?
There is no harm in this if it makes the girl happier.

What can an adolescent girl do to keep her breasts from sagging?
She should wear a brassiere that gives her breasts good support. There are no exercises that can keep the breasts from sagging if there is a familial tendency to have enlarged, sagging breasts. Of course, obesity will cause the breasts to enlarge and sag, and young girls should be encouraged to stay trim.

Is it normal for some girls to have painful breasts before the start of menstruation?

Yes. In such cases the mother should assure the child that this is normal and she should urge the girl to endure the discomfort. Otherwise, she can wear a good supporting brassiere. It is not good practice to be overly sympathetic or to medicate these children. Behavior patterns develop very early in a child's life, and if too much attention is paid to these pains, the child will tend to overemphasize them during her mature years.

Do children ever develop breast tumors?
Malignant tumors are extremely rare in immature breasts.

Should a lump be removed from the breast of a female who has not yet reached puberty?

This should not be done because what might be interpreted as a tumor is usually an enlargement of the glandular tissue. If the tissue is removed, the child will not develop a normal breast as she matures.

How can a physician distinguish between a true tumor of the breast and precocious enlargement of the gland?

A needle biopsy will tell whether there is any abnormal tumor tissue. If the report of a needle biopsy is negative, then the enlargement should be left alone. It is only when a needle biopsy gives indication of a malignancy that surgery should be undertaken.

What is the treatment for fibroadenoma of the breast in an adolescent?

A simple excision of the tumor through a small incision is all that is necessary.

Is a fibroadenoma in an adolescent a sign of a glandular upset?

No. The cause of these tumors is completely unknown.

Why should a fibroadenoma be treated at all?

Because such tumors have a tendency to enlarge. Moreover, one cannot always be absolutely certain of the nature of the tumor unless it is removed and examined microscopically.

Do fibroadenomas tend to recur?

No, but a new one in another part of the breast may develop.

Is enlargement of the nipple ever seen in little girls?

Yes, this is a rare condition, but it is occasionally seen during the first three years of life. In some cases there may be enlargement of one side only.

How long does it take from the onset of breast development until the breast has matured to its full growth potential?

This is a process that takes about three to four years. The breast will start to grow anywhere from the tenth to the twelfth year, but will not attain its full maturity until the fifteenth or sixteenth year.

Can harm result from an adolescent girl not wearing a brassiere?

No. Young breasts do not really require the protection of a brassiere.

6 HAIR

Many husbands and lovers would like to say to their women, "Why don't you get rid of the hair on your breasts?" Instead, they accept the hair as a nonremediable phenomenon or refrain from comment for the same reasons that one might hesitate to tell a loved one of his or her bad breath.

There is a great variation in the amount of hair that women have on their breasts. Some women have no hair at all whereas others have a great amount of hair around the nipples and on the surrounding skin. Distribution of hair in this area is simply an inherited characteristic and a woman can do nothing to avoid it. Generally, lighter complexioned women have no hair or less hair on the breasts, or at least they seem to have less because of the light color of the growth.

Unsightly breast hair is unnecessary, as it can be cut, plucked, shaved, or removed through electrolysis. There is a rather generally accepted but erroneous notion that hair grows in thicker and in greater abundance if it is cut or shaved. This is not true. Shaving or cutting hair on the breast is a harmless procedure, not followed by any increase in thickness or quantity of growth.

Hair also grows in greater or lesser amounts on a woman's chest wall between the breasts. This, too, can be removed without untoward results by cutting, shaving, or electrolysis.

The amount of hair a woman has on her breasts or chest wall is seldom associated with an upset in glandular function or any other underlying defect. Of course, if for one reason or another, a woman is given large doses of male sex hormones for any length of time, hair will grow where it has never grown before. Also, if a woman has a tumor of the ovary or adrenal glands, she may grow excess hair on the chest and breasts.

Electrolysis for the destruction of breast or chest wall hair is a simple, safe, effective, albeit painful, procedure. It can be readily carried out for any woman who is self-conscious about the hair and wants it removed. When performed by a competent, licensed electrologist, hair seldom grows back. If it does, it can be treated again with an electric needle.

Questions and Answers

Why is it that some women have hair around their nipples and others do not?

The distribution and amount of hair on the breasts, like hair elsewhere on the body, is an inherited characteristic. If both parents' bodies show sparse hair growth, in all probability their offspring will too.

Can anything be done to prevent the growth of hair on the breast or chest wall?

No.

How often will one have to go to an electrologist to have the hair removed?

This depends entirely on the amount of hair and the woman's ability to tolerate the discomfort of electrolysis. Some patients require but one visit; others may need a dozen or more.

Does the hair usually grow back after electrolysis?

The majority of hair follicles are destroyed with the electric needle. As a consequence, results are usually permanent.

Is local anesthesia necessary when performing electrolysis?

It is not necessary if one can tolerate the pain. If the pain is not well tolerated, injections of a local anesthetic agent can be given.

How does one find a licensed electrologist?

A dermatologist (skin specialist) can recommend one. Also, they usually are listed in classified telephone directories.

Will shaving the hair on the breast cause it to grow in thicker?

No. This is an erroneous notion. However, when the returning hair is only slightly above skin level, the stubble may feel thicker. All hair is thickest at or just above skin level.

Will cutting the hair with a scissors cause it to grow in thicker?
No.

Should one safely pluck the hair around the nipples?
Yes, it can be done safely, but the hair will grow back.

Will the taking of oral contraceptive pills or estrogen cause hair to grow on the breast?
No.

Does the downy hair that grows on the breast of adolescent girls tend to disappear when maturity is reached?
Much of it does disappear.

Is it safe to bleach the hair on the breast or chest wall?
Yes.

Is there a tendency for an increased growth of hair on the breast after change of life?
Usually not.

Will the taking of hormones for the symptoms of change of life cause hair to grow on the breast?
No. Although some of the medications given may contain small quantities of male sex hormone, the amount is insufficient to stimulate growth of hair.

7 BRASSIERES

In ancient art the breast was sculptured or painted in its bare state, or covered only by a thin drape or toga. In Western civilization the undergarment, including the brassiere, did not come into being until the medieval era, when religious teachings began to insist on modesty and the coverup of the female nude. But the brassiere had purposes more important than shielding the breast from view: it molded and beautified the breasts by rounding out their contours, and it supported them when they were heavy and pendulous.

Within recent times, with the long overdue emancipation of the female in all areas of human activity, the brassiere has come under attack. Many women, especially the younger ones, resent the physical inhibitions brought about by the wearing of a brassiere when it serves no purpose in supporting a structure capable of self-support. Others have abandoned the bra in defiance of the male-inspired edict that it is "proper" to wear one.

Physicians are frequently asked whether it is harmful to go without a brassiere. The answer is no. True, it may be uncomfortable or even painful if the breast is heavy and pendulous, but no real physical damage will result from bralessness.

Full- and heavy-breasted women usually wear uplift brassieres, and it is surprising how many of them are poorly constructed and fitted. Some —in an attempt to make the breast appear smaller—are so tight that they inhibit normal breathing; others are so loose that they lend little or no support; and still others have straps that are so narrow that they dig into and cause irritation of the skin at the shoulders.

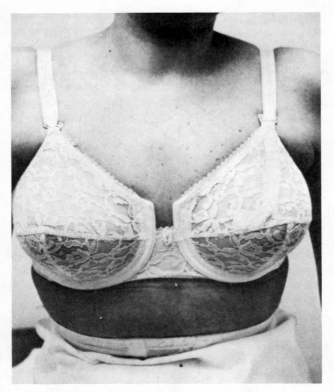

A good uplift brassiere should be worn by all women who have large breasts.

Small-breasted women often use brassieres that are padded in various ways to make the bust seem larger or more elevated. These contraptions are, of course, harmless and frequently benefit a woman's ego. As we know, some bras contain metal stays that help support the breasts or in other ways improve contours. From a medical point of view, there is no harm from the metal unless it creates undue pressure on the breast and chest wall. Every once in a while one encounters a patient with a crescent-shaped lumpiness in the under portion of the breast where the metal of a brassiere has exerted too much pressure on the fat tissue for too long a period of time. Patients with such lumps are fearful that they have developed a tumor. In reality, neither tumors nor cancers result from brassieres. However, the pressure from the metal may cause some of the fat beneath the skin to be replaced by fibrous tissue (fibrosis) within the fat tissue of the breast, thus causing it to feel thick and tumorlike.

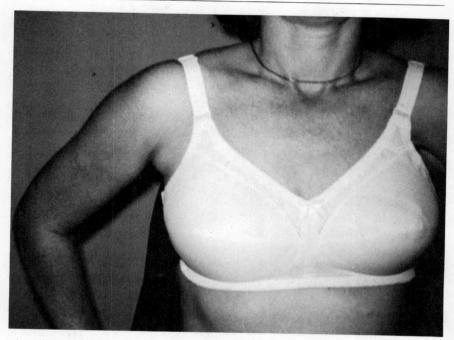

A well-fitted brassiere will hide the fact that a patient has had a breast removed. This woman has undergone a left mastectomy.

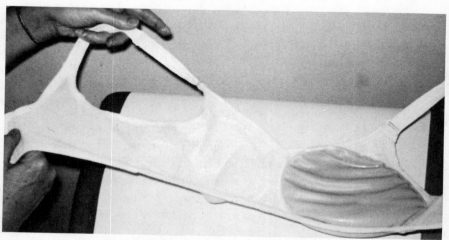

A postmastectomy brassiere is specially constructed so that a plastic sac, filled with fluid, can fit into the empty cup.

Sometimes the shoulder straps or underbust band of a brassiere makes contact with a mole on the front or back of the chest wall, or on the shoulders. As the brassiere shifts innumerable times during the course of a woman's activities, repeated friction may be placed on the mole. If continued over a period of years, such irritation may cause an innocent, harmless mole to change color, grow, or bleed. In some instances the mole may undergo malignant degeneration. To avoid this, it is recommended that a mole subjected to constant irritation from any part of a brassiere should be removed prophylactically.

During pregnancy it is important that the breasts receive proper support because of their enlargement. A specially designed brassiere should be purchased during the early months of pregnancy, preferably one that is adjustable so that it can be let out as pregnancy progresses. Special nursing bras are available for women who are breast-feeding their infants.

Another special bra is for after breast removal, when patients are anxious to obtain a brassiere that will restore the outward appearance of the bust, even in an evening gown or bathing suit. These can be purchased and worn as soon as the surgical wound has healed, usually within a matter of two weeks after surgery. The cup on the affected side is supplied with a plastic sac filled with a fluid that has the consistency of breast tissue. If one feels the chest area through the clothing, it may not be possible to tell on which side the breast has been removed.

The Consumer Service Division of the International Ladies Garment Workers Union has issued a useful pamphlet on how to determine the correct size of a brassiere, and the instructions are reprinted below:

HOW TO DETERMINE YOUR CORRECT BRA SIZE:

To do this, you will need a tape measure. Put it around your rib cage, under the bust—take a snug, not a tight measurement. Then add 5″ to this measurement for your correct size. For example: if your underbust measurement is 29″, add 5 and your size is 34. If this measurement turns out to be an in-between size (for instance 35″) try on both a size 34 and a 36 and judge which gives you the best fit.

To determine your correct CUP size: Measure around the bust at its fullest. If this measurement is identical to your bra size, the cup you will require is an A. If the measurement is one inch more than the bra size, the cup is B. Two inches over is a C; three inches over a D.

WAYS TO CHECK FOR CORRECT FIT:

- Be sure it stays close to your body, that there are no gaps between the cups.

- If the breasts are forced toward the sides or center, the cup is too small.

- If the cup is not filled out, a smaller or foam-lined cup may be needed. If flesh overflows, a larger cup or a style with more coverage is necessary.

- Check the underbust band. It should fit snugly, not tightly. If it rides up, it's too tight. If you can run your finger easily under the band, the fit is correct.

- Check the back. If it rides up, the fit around your body is too tight.

Questions and Answers

At what age should a girl be permitted to wear a brassiere?

Whenever she wants to, regardless of age. If her friends wear brassieres, there is no harm to a child without much breast development wearing one. The harm arises when a squabble develops in the family over the issue.

Is it safe to tape one's breasts in order to make them appear more upright?

Yes, provided one is not allergic or sensitive to the adhesive in the tape.

How does one know whether she is wearing a properly fitting brassiere?

See method of fitting, in the text of this chapter.

Should women have brassieres of more than one size?

Yes, if their breasts swell prior to menstruation. When such swelling is marked, it may require a larger brassiere.

Should women with inordinately heavy breasts wear broad shoulder straps on their brassieres?

Yes, otherwise the straps will press into the shoulders and produce irritation and pain.

Are uplift brassieres always necessary?

No. Some women have naturally high-positioned breasts.

Will wearing an uplift brassiere for a number of years cause the breasts to be firmer and higher on the chest wall?

No.

Will the continued wearing of an uplift brassiere prevent a breast from becoming flat and pendulous?

Usually not. However, if a breast is very heavy and already sags, it may prevent further stretching of the fibers that help hold it up.

Should a woman wear a brassiere 24 hours a day if she has painful breasts?

Yes, if it helps reduce her pain. Unfortunately, painful breasts may not necessarily be relieved by wearing a brassiere.

Will wearing a brassiere 24 hours a day help pregnant women whose breasts are painful?

Yes, in some instances.

Is it wise for a woman who has just undergone minor breast surgery to wear a brassiere 24 hours a day?

Patients with large breasts usually find the wound area to be less painful if they wear a brassiere continually.

Can harm result from wearing strapless brassieres?

No.

Are women ever allergic to the materials from which brassieres are made?

Yes, especially when synthetic materials are used.

Are there any harmful effects from brassieres with cutout nipples?
No.

8 PREGNANCY AND THE BREAST

The breast reacts to the onset of pregnancy within a week or two after conception. Many women who have had previous pregnancies are able to diagnose another pregnancy by virtue of their breasts continuing to feel full and heavy after their would-be period has passed. Doctors, too, can make a diagnosis of pregnancy in some patients merely by feeling the rubbery fullness of the breasts, which comes on within two to three weeks after a skipped menstrual period. We have seen in an earlier chapter how these changes arise because of the increased amount of hormones that circulate in the blood following the onset of pregnancy.

As pregnancy proceeds, breast enlargement and fullness continue, but a tenderness, experienced at first, disappears. Toward the middle of pregnancy, the characteristic increase in the amount of pigment in the nipple is noted and the small Montgomery glands within the nipple become prominent. Blonde women with pink nipples may note a change in nipples to light brown; brunettes and blacks may find their nipples changed to a very dark brown or brownish black. The reason for these pigment changes is not known. After childbirth, the color of the nipples may lighten somewhat but they do not usually change back to their prepregnant tint.

Although pregnancy does cause the breast to lose some of its rounded, conical shape, in many women this change is minimal. If the woman remains thin during the pregnancy and wears a good supporting brassiere, her breasts should not change significantly. The trouble is that too many pregnant women gain too much weight and permit their breasts to get inordinately heavy. This may lead to persistent sagging after the pregnancy is completed.

Because the pregnant breast is engorged and slightly more tender than the nonpregnant gland, it must be safeguarded against possible injury. This does not mean that a woman must exclude her breasts from their usual participation in the sex act, but it should dictate a certain amount of restraint on the part of the mate.

Inverted nipples present a problem to a woman who wants to nurse her child. Repeated massage and manipulation throughout pregnancy has little or no beneficial effect. The only hope of everting the nipples is to subject them to the suckling action of the newborn infant. In some cases, eversion through nursing is sufficient to permit successful breast-feeding; in other instances, it fails.

During the latter half of pregnancy, the breasts may discharge a few drops of a clear or milky liquid, or, on rare occasions, a drop or two of blood. These are all normal phenomena and should cause no alarm. Nipple discharge is merely a reflection of the increased activity within the glands and ducts of the breast as it readies itself for lactation. And of course, immediately prior to and for a day or two after childbirth the breast secretes colostrum, the thick, yellowish gray substance that is the forerunner of milk, and which has a high protein content.

The breast during pregnancy may develop a cyst, a benign tumor, and in rare instances, a cancer. Cysts and benign solid tumors are no more likely to occur during pregnancy than at other times. If the pregnancy is well advanced, these lesions can be safely ignored until several weeks after childbirth. If they grow to sizable proportions during early pregnancy, they should be removed surgically.

The cancer affecting the pregnant breast is called inflammatory cancer because the condition is accompanied by marked swelling, redness, heat, and tenderness. Fortunately, this is an extremely rare disease, as the ultimate cure of this particular kind of cancer is most difficult to obtain. Surgical removal of the breast is indicated as soon as a positive diagnosis has been made. With the earlier recognition of this type of breast cancer within recent years, and with radical surgery, five-year survival rates have increased from 15 percent in 1940 to approximately 35–40 percent today.

Questions and Answers

Should pregnant women rub their breasts with special creams or cocoa butter to prevent stretch lines from forming?

In all probability, these measures are of no value in preventing stretch lines. The best way to avoid them is not to get too fat during pregnancy.

What creams can be used for the nipples?

In all probability, creams are unnecessary. However, some obstetricians advise the use of Mammal cream or Massé cream for the nipples.

Are the breasts more prone to injury during pregnancy?

Only insofar as they are larger. Also, since they are more tender, an injury will be more painful than ordinarily.

Will vigorous physical exercise damage the pregnant breast?
No.

Is it safe for a pregnant woman to permit manipulation of her breasts during pregnancy?

Yes. Alterations in one's usual sex habits are unnecessary until the last two months of pregnancy.

Do the breasts ever enlarge abnormally during pregnancy?

Yes, hypertrophy may ensue. However, this is an extremely rare condition. When it does occur, it may involve both breasts or only one breast.

What is the treatment for inverted nipples during pregnancy?

Little can be done for them although the creams, mentioned above, might sometimes prove helpful. The best treatment will be the suction created by the nursing infant.

Should pregnant women who plan to nurse their children express colostrum and attempt to "toughen" the nipples during the last stages of pregnancy?

No. They should leave them alone.

Is there a greater tendency for a cyst to form during pregnancy than at other times?

Only slightly greater, as milk cysts (galactoceles) occasionally arise from a blocked milk duct.

How successful is treatment for breast cancer occurring during pregnancy?

Not as successful as treatment during other times.

If a pregnant woman learns that she has breast cancer will the pregnancy have to be terminated?

Not necessarily, especially if it is in the later months of the pregnancy.

9 BREAST-FEEDING

The resurgence of natural childbirth in this country after a lapse of some one hundred years has brought along with it renewed interest in breast-feeding. Young women who select natural childbirth as their form of delivery appear to be especially concerned about all the experiences they and their newborns will undergo during and after the pregnancy, and they often decide to nurse their children. Estimates are that breast-feeding has increased threefold in the past twenty-five years, even though bottle-feeding is still the method most American women choose for their young.

Most obstetricians and pediatricians agree that it is somewhat better for the child's health if the mother decides to nurse the infant. This presupposes that the mother is in robust health and will not be too exhausted by the extra demands placed upon her by breast-feeding. It assumes that her breasts are normal and capable of nursing. Also, it assumes that the newborn is at full term and is physically healthy. Premature babies, exceptionally weak babies, infants born with jaundice, and those with defects such as harelip or cleft palate are better off bottle fed.

Despite the preference a doctor may have for natural feeding, he seldom pushes his belief upon his patient. He knows full well that the infant's health can be maintained adequately with bottle-feeding.

The preference for breast-feeding is based on the fact that mother's milk has all the right components for the baby's growth and development. Moreover, mother's milk is the proper temperature, it is sterile and pure, and contains many immune substances to help protect the child against disease.

Women who feel no obligation to breast-feed their infant should not be subjected to a sense of guilt. They should be assured by their doctor that the child will not suffer physically from bottle-feeding and will grow up to love her just the same, as though he never missed the experience of nursing at the breast. Much has been said recently about a sense of deprivation that the infant might feel when he is forced to substitute a bottle for a breast. If such a feeling exists, it can be eliminated easily by cuddling and caressing the child during and after the feeding period. It should be kept in mind that a mother who has strong feelings against nursing may become tense and irritable if she is forced to do so. Then, instead of developing a closer, warmer feeling toward her infant, she may develop resentment that will damage the relationship far more than breast-feeding can bind it.

Some women elect to nurse their children not out of a true desire to do so but because of a fear that they may one day develop breast cancer if they fail to nurse. There is no positive proof that breast cancer is greatly influenced by nursing or nonnursing, except that there is less incidence of this disease in countries where breast-feeding is the general custom. In this regard, it should be mentioned that certain types of cancer are more prevalent than others among certain races because of genetic factors. Thus, Orientals have a lower incidence of breast cancer but a higher incidence of stomach cancer than Caucasians.

There are many other factors that must govern a woman's decision to breast-feed or not to breast-feed an infant. A woman with markedly inverted nipples may be unable to nurse; a woman who is particularly anxious to retain the youthful appearance of her breasts may not want to nurse; an infant may reject its mother's milk or may obtain insufficient quantities to sustain it; a mother may work and therefore not be available to nurse the infant; the birth of twins or triplets may result in an inadequate milk supply from the breasts; and so on. Whatever the factors motivating the decision not to nurse, the mother should rest assured that her infant will not suffer.

And there is still the question of cosmetics. There is little doubt that pregnancy itself may produce a flattening of the breast, but nursing is something else again. Women who have never given birth to a child tend to retain a more rounded, upright appearance to their breasts; women who have had several children tend to have breasts that are flatter and sag more than those who have given birth to but one child; and breasts that have nursed several children sag and flatten out more than those that have never nursed. The significance of these changes to a woman can be measured by her vanity or lack thereof.

Questions and Answers

How soon after the child is born is it put to the mother's breast?
Within approximately twelve hours.

Should a mother alternate the breasts that she offers to her child?
Yes.

Are all women capable of supplying sufficient milk to adequately nourish their newborn children?
Most are, but some may have a sparse supply. In these cases, supplemental bottles of cow's milk are given.

How long a period should a child be allowed to nurse?
This varies greatly from child to child. Some take all they want in five minutes; slow feeders may take twenty minutes.

What special care should be given to the nipples during the nursing period?
Cleanliness is the most important objective. The nipples should be washed with ordinary soap and water before and after each nursing. A comfortable, well-fitting, uplift brassiere should be worn.

Is it permissible for a mother to take pain-relieving medications when she stops nursing?
Yes.

Can any permanent harm result to the breasts from nursing?
No. Nature intended them primarily for just that purpose.

Are there special nursing brassieres?
Yes. They open up the front and allow for the easy exposure of the breast without requiring the mother to disrobe.

Should a nursing mother wear a brassiere 24 hours a day?

Not necessarily. If it makes her feel more comfortable, then she should do it.

How can a mother tell if her breast is not supplying the baby with enough milk?

She will learn this very quickly as the infant will evidence his dissatisfaction by crying for more milk.

What can be done if a mother must be away from the child for two or three days during the nursing period?

She should be sure to empty her breasts at regular intervals so that caking does not take place and so that her breasts are continually stimulated to produce milk. She can do this manually at regular intervals, or use a breast pump.

Should a mother who is breast-feeding her child empty her breasts manually even if she skips one nursing day?

Yes.

Will a breast continue to secrete milk after a child stops nursing?

It usually takes about a week for the breasts to dry up. Every once in a while a woman will continue to secrete milk indefinitely, even though she has stopped nursing.

Will the normal breast continue to give milk so long as the child nurses?

In most women, yes. Occasionally, the supply dwindles after several months of nursing.

Do the breasts usually return to normal size after the nursing period has ended?

Yes, but they may flatten out to a lesser or greater degree, and some sagging may ensue.

Does the baby's suckling accelerate the flow of milk?

Yes.

Can a mother resume nursing if she has omitted several days?
Yes, but the milk flow may not be adequate unless the breasts are emptied at regular intervals.

Can a woman whose breasts have caked resume nursing?
Yes, but it is not always followed by a satisfactory milk flow.

Will caking of the breast disappear spontaneously?
Yes, within a few days.

What is the treatment for caked breasts?
Warm compresses and pain-relieving medications. The breasts should be supported by a brassiere.

To avoid cracked nipples, should soap not be used in cleansing the breasts?
Soap may be conducive to the development of cracked nipples. Consequently, it is probably best to clean the nipples with a mild cleansing cream and to apply substances such as Mammal cream or Massé cream.

Is the use of cocoa butter helpful in avoiding cracked nipples?
Yes, to a limited extent.

What is the treatment for cracked nipples?
1. A specially designed nipple shield should be used. This will enable the infant to nurse by suckling a rubber nipple. The suction created by the infant will cause the milk to flow, but there will be no direct contact between the breast and the mouth.
2. A healing ointment, such as Mammal cream or Massé cream, can be applied to the nipple.
3. The mother should avoid the use of soap when she cleanses the nipple area. Warm water is sufficient.
4. A good, snug brassiere should be worn.

Do some newborns reject mother's milk but accept cow's milk?
Yes, this happens occasionally. Also, a child can sometimes be allergic to its mother's milk but not to cow's milk.

Is there benefit from nursing during the first day or two before the milk comes in?

Yes. First of all, nursing will stimulate the milk flow. Secondly, the infant will obtain colostrum from nursing. This substance is rich in proteins and is thought to contain large quantities of beneficial antibodies that will help to ward off infection during the first days of life. Soon afterward, the infant develops his own antibodies to protect against bacteria and viruses.

Will the milk dry up spontaneously if the mother doesn't nurse?

The breasts will dry up, but caking with marked tenderness, pain, and swelling will develop.

What is done to prevent caking and to dry up the breasts if the mother decides not to nurse?

1. At the time of delivery an injection is given to the mother that will control the situation. It is a hormone known as Deladumone, or

2. The obstetrician will prescribe stilbestrol tablets for a few days. This will have the same effect as the Deladumone.

Is there any harm in giving hormones to dry up the breasts?
No.

Is it necessary to give hormones to dry up the breasts when the mother has weaned her child?

Usually not. When a mother stops nursing after several months, the breasts ordinarily dry up spontaneously.

Are the breasts more likely to develop milk cysts if a mother does not nurse?

Yes, but the condition is not encountered very frequently. It should be remembered that a breast is meant to nurse, and that milk cysts, as well as other abnormal conditions, may arise if the breast fails to fulfill its function.

What is the treatment for a galactocele (milk cyst)?

Usually galactoceles subside spontaneously, but if one doesn't, surgical excision is indicated.

Should a mother stop nursing if she has infection in her breast?

Not necessarily. With the judicious use of appropriate antibiotic medications a good number of breast infections can be overcome while the infant continues to nurse. Naturally, if a surgical incision and drainage of a breast abscess is necessary, nursing must be abandoned.

Is it permissible to resume breast-feeding after an inflammation or infection has subsided?

Yes, but the milk flow may stop if the child is removed from the breast for too long a time.

Is it often necessary to operate on an infection that develops during the nursing period?

This will depend on the susceptibility of the bacteria to the antibiotic being administered. If the bacteria causing the infection are not sensitive to the antibiotic, an abscess requiring surgery may develop.

Do premature babies do better by being artificially fed?

Yes, since their ability to nurse may be quite limited. It takes considerable muscle strength for any newborn to suckle a breast successfully.

Can a mother satisfactorily nurse twins or triplets?

Yes, but in the majority of cases, the breast-feedings require supplementation with cow's milk.

What foods should a nursing mother be sure to include in her diet?

A full, regular diet with the usual amounts of protein, carbohydrates, and fat should be eaten. Salads and fruits are to be included in such a diet.

Are there certain foods that a nursing mother must avoid?

No. As she proceeds with nursing, however, she may discover that her infant rejects her milk when she has eaten certain foods. In that event, she should omit that item from her diet. She should also be sure to drink plenty of fluids, including three to four glasses of milk a day.

What type of vitamins and minerals should a nursing mother take?

She should continue with the same multivitamin tablets, fortified with minerals, that she had been taking during her pregnancy.

Should a nursing mother avoid spicy and highly seasoned foods?
No.

Will drinking large amounts of alcohol or smoking to excess adversely affect the nursing mother's milk?
It might not directly affect the milk, but a mother who drinks to excess often does not eat a well-balanced diet. Tobacco is especially bad if the mother smokes while nursing.

Should a nursing mother get additional rest?
Yes. It is a demanding effort to nurse a newborn and therefore she requires extra rest periods.

Do tensions and anxieties affect a mother's milk?
Not directly, but it is amazing how even an infant seems to know when its nursing mother is especially upset.

Can a nursing mother's medications affect her milk?
Barbiturates, taken in large doses, may be transmitted through the mother's milk and may make a child drowsy. Certain laxatives, if taken regularly and in large amounts, may cause the nursing infant to have loose stools.

Do nursing children contract disease through mother's milk?
No, but some physicians think that a mother who is allergic may cause her nursing child to become sensitive to certain allergens to which she is sensitive.

For how long a period should the average child be breast-fed?
As long as the mother wishes to, and as long as the child wants to breast-feed. Naturally, when the child has reached six months to one year of age, he is on solid foods and relies much less on milk for gratification of his hunger. He may then show less interest in breast-feeding and more interest in other forms of sustenance.

Will it hurt a child if the mother decides to discontinue nursing after two, three, or four months?
No. If weaned properly, most children readily accept a bottle instead of a breast.

Should an infant be weaned from the breast gradually?

Yes. This comes about without too much fuss as infants sleep the night through when they reach a few months of age and therefore become accustomed to missing breast-feeding. Also, they readily accept solid and semisolid foods as a substitute for breast-feeding.

What should the mother do after she stops nursing?

She should wear a firmly fitting brassiere or binder on her breasts. She should also limit her fluid intake for several days. If the breasts are not emptied periodically they will not refill, as the greatest impetus for milk formation is the periodic suckling process.

Should a nursing mother permit her breasts to be stimulated during marital relations?

There is no harm in the practice but it may stimulate milk flow.

Will the breasts continue to secrete milk if they are manipulated and suckled during lovemaking following the nursing period?

Yes, if it happens regularly.

Will breast-feeding increase the chances of developing a tumor or cancer of the breast?

No.

10 THE BREAST AS A SEX ORGAN

The breast is a secondary sex organ in that it is not essential for the process of reproduction. However, from early childhood throughout all of life, the female considers the breast to be a primary emblem of her sexuality. In fact, the breast is the only visible, apparent female sex organ known to a young girl. It is not until she reaches older childhood or attains puberty that she learns the anatomy of her genitals and realizes that she is as well equipped as the male even though her organs are internally located. Until then, little girls who see the genitals of brothers or other boys may feel somewhat deprived and envious. Their envy is relieved to a certain extent when they begin to appreciate that the breast is their special endowment. Then, when adolescence progresses, they actually swell with pride and display their "sexiness" through their breasts.

The female breast is well constructed anatomically to serve as a sex organ. There are special nerve endings in the nipple that are capable of receiving and sending erotic sensations. The nipple is composed of so-called erogenous tissue (as is the penis) with tiny muscle fibers that can contract and cause the nipple to become erect on sexual manipulation and stimulation. Although when the nipple is suckled by a nursing infant it also becomes erect, the mother does not experience truly erotic sensations.

The breast is extremely important in the developing life of every young girl as it is generally involved in the earliest sexual contacts. As she shows signs of development, she discovers that boys want to touch her breasts and that when they do, she becomes sexually aroused. Manipulation or kissing the breast not only causes the nipple to become firm and erect but the pulse quickens, respirations increase, and the glands in the vulva and vagina begin to secrete mucus. These responses are present to a greater or lesser degree, depending on the sensitivity of the individual and her desire or lack of desire to engage in sexual activity.

In discussing this subject, it is interesting to note that some girls and young women have strong inhibitions about permitting themselves to be touched or kissed on the breasts. Some have an actual aversion toward breast stimulation. These reactions can sometimes be attributed to parental admonitions during childhood and early adolescence that there are "dangers" in permitting a boy to touch or kiss a girl's breast. Other inhibitions stem from a girl's fear that the inevitable excitement following breast stimulation will cause her to lose control of herself to such an extent that she will engage in all-out sexual relations. Still other females harbor the erroneous notion that repeated manipulation or suckling will result in actual physical injury, causing the breasts to lose their firmness or even to develop cancer later on in life.

Reluctance to permit the breasts to play a significant role in lovemaking frequently stems from a woman's lack of pride in the appearance of her breasts. Of course, here one should exclude the frigid woman who derives little or no pleasure from any type of sexual stimulation, whether it be breast, clitoral, or vaginal in nature. In this discussion, we are dealing with women who are otherwise sexually active and who enjoy intercourse and reach satisfactory climaxes despite the fact that they do not engage in foreplay involving breast stimulation.

Even in homosexual relations between females, the breasts often play a part quite similar to that which prevails in the most natural of heterosexual relations. The one who acts out the role of aggressor frequently manipulates and stimulates the other's breasts as if she were a male. Not infrequently a homosexual female will reach a climax when her girl friend caresses and kisses her breasts, but will feel no sensual pleasure when a man stimulates them in the same manner.

Listed below are the types of some of the more common reasons why they might want to exclude the breast from foreplay prior to intercourse:

1. Women with inverted nipples, who receive no pleasurable sensation from nipple manipulation or suckling.

2. Women with exceptionally large, pendulous breasts, who are ashamed of their "deformity."

3. Women who may be ashamed of a marked asymmetry of the breasts.

4. Women with exceptionally small breasts, who may fear their mate will think their breasts inadequate.

5. Women whose breasts are extremely sensitive and who reach climax quickly upon breast stimulation. The number of women in this category is not great. Most are young, and as they mature, they learn to control their orgasms.

6. Women who have undergone plastic surgery and have visible scars. Some women who have received implants to enlarge their breasts may fear that vigorous stimulation will disrupt the implant; others do not want their lovers to discover that they have had breast-augmentation surgery.

7. Women who have undergone breast removal frequently want to avoid their mate's contact with the remaining breast. However, experience shows that a mate will adjust very quickly to his wife's condition and if he enjoyed caressing the breasts prior to mastectomy, he will continue to enjoy contact with the remaining breast.

Although it may seem elementary to some readers, the following medical facts concerning breasts and their role in sex activity should be recorded:

1. Breast manipulation and suckling are natural components of the sex act. By stimulating her desire and by causing vaginal secretions, it prepares the female for subsequent intercourse.

2. Some females are not aroused to intercourse without a preceding period of breast stimulation. Moreover, breast stimulation will often quicken the female climax to coincide with a more aroused mate.

3. Prolonged stimulation of the breasts sometimes causes the male to become so aroused that he ejaculates soon after entrance. (Repeated sexual contacts over a period of weeks or months will usually overcome this tendency.)

4. Some females are so sensitive that prolonged breast stimulation will cause them to reach orgasm before the male has initiated intercourse. (Repeated contacts should make it possible for the male to know just how much pre-intercourse breast stimulation should be engaged in.)

5. The size of a woman's nipples or breasts is not a gauge of their sensitivity nor of her reaction to stimulation. Some large breasts may be nonreactive whereas some small breasts can be extremely sensitive.

6. Females who find breast stimulation distasteful should discuss their reactions with their husbands. If it is found that the reaction interferes with full enjoyment of sexual relations, the matter should be discussed with a physician. In most instances, the aversion toward breast stimulation is psychological in origin. Those women who think their breasts are ugly, and therefore shield them from their mates, should also consult a physician who might be able to tell them how to improve the appearance of their breasts. Loss of weight in stout women, gain of weight in thin women, removal of hair about the nipples, may accomplish this. In others, plastic surgery on the breasts may be advisable.

A man must be considerate toward the woman who is reluctant to permit her breasts to play a part in sexual activity. If he insists, against her will, upon actively stimulating the breasts he may encounter a frigid reaction when he commences actual intercourse.

7. Breasts are usually tender, especially the outer portions, just before menstruation. It is important therefore for the man to be particularly gentle during this period.

8. Some people enjoy contacts between the breasts and the male genitals. This is a natural urge and should be satisfied if both parties are agreeable. If the woman finds the practice distasteful, she should discuss it openly with her mate. (It is always better to engage in sex practices that are desired by *both* parties.)

9. If a man desires to resume lovemaking after his wife has already had a climax, breast stimulation is often a good method of rearousing her.

10. After childbirth and nursing, the breast should return to a fully resting state before it is again stimulated by the husband. Strong manipulation may injure the gland tissue or ducts in a breast that is, or has just recently completed, nursing. Repeated suckling of such a breast may continue the flow of milk for an almost indefinite period.

11. Although the breast area can be hurt by biting the nipples, or by squeezing, pinching, or sucking too hard, it will not cause a tumor or cancer to grow. As in all other aspects of the love act, the male should be motivated by an affectionate, gentle attitude. A violent man is not necessarily a good lover, and he may cause real damage to the fat tissue in the breast by pinching or squeezing too hard. An infection or abscess can be the result of uncontrolled sucking or biting.

Questions and Answers

What is the value of a mother's alerting her adolescent daughter to the consequences of breast stimulation?

In some areas of society it may seem old fashioned but it is surprising how often physicians are asked about possible harmful effects from breast stimulation. Girls should not be made to feel that this type of contact is "dirty," "wrong," or abnormal, as such misinformation may create an unnecessary sense of guilt. The majority of adolescents participate in this form of loveplay and it is unwise to make them think they are unique. Actually, the breast is the first target of activity after sex awakening. If a child is made to think she is sinning by allowing a boy to touch her breasts, it may lead to neurotic sexual behavior when she matures. Children should *never* be misled into thinking that breast stimulation might lead to the future development of cancer!

What percentage of people indulge in breast stimulation as a foreplay to intercourse?

It is estimated that well over 98 percent do.

Do some women desire breast stimulation during intercourse?

Yes. There are women who cannot reach a climax unless the breast is vigorously stimulated during intercourse. This can be accomplished most easily when the female straddles the male.

Does desire for breast stimulation vary from time to time?

Yes. Some women may enjoy this activity except for the two to three days prior to menstruation when the breast may be so swollen and tender as to make breast stimulation painful. Other women dislike breast stimulation during pregnancy, or during the time they are nursing a child.

Sexual appetite varies during different periods of a woman's life and, for no known reason, a woman who has enjoyed breast stimulation at one time may dislike it at other times. These variations are normal, and reflect changes in the psychological attitudes of people toward their mates. A woman who bears hostility toward her husband may still permit him to have intercourse because she feels it is her duty to do so, but she may refuse him when he attempts to fondle or kiss her breasts. To some women, breast stimulation is every bit as intimate an act as intercourse itself.

Are the breasts ever inadvertently injured during loveplay?

This sometimes occurs because the woman is so excited that she does not feel the hurt of excessive stimulation. Then, when relations have ended, she becomes aware that the breast has been injured.

Do some women derive pleasure when their breasts are bitten and excessively stimulated?

Yes. This is a form of neurotic behavior known as masochism. In some cases, climax can be achieved only when they are injured or beaten.

Is there a wide variation in reactions to breast stimulation?

Yes. Some women may approach climax when their breasts are manipulated and kissed; others have no response whatever from vigorous breast stimulation.

Should a woman perfume her breasts prior to going to bed with her mate?

Men do find certain scents sexually stimulating, but women should place the perfume between or under the breasts, not on the nipples. No matter how exciting the scent, perfume will not taste good when placed on the nipples. Also, perfume has an alcohol base, and may burn the delicate tissues of the nipples.

Do some women desire contact between their breasts and the male genitals?

Yes. This is a normal sexual response.

Is it abnormal if a woman reaches a climax by contact between her breasts and the male genitals?

No. Most physicians believe that any sexual practice that gives pleasure to both parties is normal for them. The practice of sexual contact between the breasts and the male genitals is often practiced, but climax is not the usual outcome.

Should women try to hide their breasts from their mates?

No. This is abnormal conduct. If two people enjoy each other's bodies and are in love, they should be frank and open about sex. A woman may not have beautiful breasts but her mate may think that they are if he loves her. (I had a patient who insisted upon wearing a brassiere during intercourse because she did not want her husband to see her pendulous, oversized breasts. When he convinced her to abandon the practice, their relations improved greatly.)

Does hair on the breasts repel some men?

Yes. Some men avoid breast stimulation as a foreplay to intercourse because they find breast hair so unattractive. (See chapter 6.)

Do some women lose interest in breast stimulation as they grow older?

Some do; others don't. Generally, if a woman desires sex as she grows older, she will continue to want her breasts caressed.

Must breast stimulation be curtailed during pregnancy?

Not until the last two or three months of pregnancy when the breasts become engorged and tender. However, the pregnant breast should be treated with greater tenderness than usual.

Should the breasts be stimulated by the husband during the period when the mother is nursing the child?

No. In addition to this being unwise from a medical point of view, women rarely wish to have their breasts stimulated sexually while they are still nursing their child.

How soon after a woman has weaned her child can her husband resume stimulation and suckling of the breasts?

It is best for him to wait until a few weeks after nursing has been discontinued. Otherwise, his activity may cause the breast to continue to secrete milk.

Is it natural for women to continue to like breast stimulation after menopause?

Yes. Most studies show that there is only a slight decrease in a woman's sexual desires after menopause. If she enjoyed breast stimulation prior to change of life, she will continue to enjoy it afterward.

Do women of menopausal age ever find breast stimulation painful?

Yes. The nipples may become very sensitive when they reach the menopausal years and even if they enjoy breast stimulation, it becomes too painful to permit.

Can a woman who has had plastic surgery on a breast enjoy breast stimulation?

Yes, the sensations are not altered by the surgery.

Will a woman still have erotic sensations from breast stimulation after she has had a plastic implant to make her breast larger?

Yes, because the implant is placed on the chest wall beneath the breast tissue and the sensations of the nipple are usually not disturbed in the performance of this operation.

11 THE BREAST DURING AND AFTER MENOPAUSE

Since it is common for the American woman to live into her mid-seventies, the postmenopausal period represents approximately one-third of her life-span. Menopause is a capricious phenomenon in that it creates severe symptoms in some women, and none at all in others. The difference in its effect is difficult to understand because its underlying cause is always the same. Menopause comes about as a result of the decrease, and eventual stoppage, of female sex hormone secretion (estrogen) by the ovaries. Some endocrinologists think that after menopause the adrenal glands secrete varying amounts of estrogen or a substance so similar that it cannot be distinguished from estrogen. If the adrenals produce a great deal of estrogen or an estrogenlike hormone in a particular woman, it may explain her lack of menopausal symptoms, and if they produce little, symptoms may be severe.

A detailed description of the symptoms and signs of menopause is not germane to the main subject of this book but it might be well to briefly mention some of them.

1. Menopause usually starts anywhere from forty-five to fifty years of age, with variations in onset and termination of two to three years in a minority of women.

2. Menstrual periods become irregular and the flow may become scant or unusually heavy.

3. Eventually menstruation ceases, anywhere from a few months to a few years after the onset of menopausal symptoms.

4. To a lesser or greater degree, women experience hot flashes, flushes, and break out into sweats.

5. The more nervous and tense a woman, the more likely is she to suffer severely and frequently from the symptoms described above.

6. As menopause is an evidence of the aging process, other signs of growing older may accompany it. These may include dryness of the skin, dryness of the membranes of the external genitals, with itching and irritation about the entrance to the vagina, and various changes within the breast (to be described later).

7. Some women at menopause are markedly irritable, tense, and depressed. Occasionally, emotional stability can be so upset that the woman requires psychiatric as well as hormone therapy.

The modern woman wants to be just as good-looking during and after menopause as she was during her younger years. Not the least of her concerns is her figure, including the appearance of her breasts. Happily, women no longer subscribe to the medieval concept that once the childbearing period of life ends, the woman's importance as a vital, attractive being ceases. Today, men and women alike believe that a female can be both physically and socially exciting far into her later years.

Studies of social and sexual behavior demonstrate clearly that the breast continues to play the same role after menopause as it did before. Women at and after menopause pay a great deal of attention to the appearance of their breasts, as they are conscious that these may be one of the first organs to betray signs of aging.

Although the breast may show very few outward signs of change during the late forties and early fifties, we have seen that usually there is a decrease in the amount of gland tissue and an increase in the amount of fibrous, inert connective tissue; also, a loss of fat tissue that causes the breast to lose some of its former rounded contour, a loss of breast skin elasticity with continued aging, and wrinkling. Lastly, the bands of fibrous

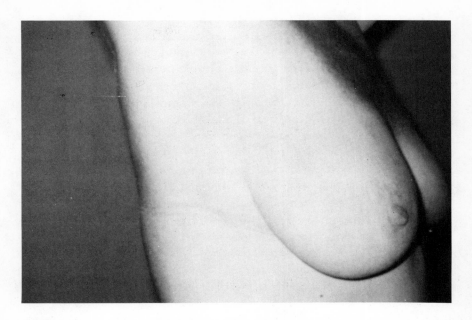

The breast does not necessarily show marked changes as a result of menopause. This 58-year-old woman has retained much of the youthful appearance of her breasts.

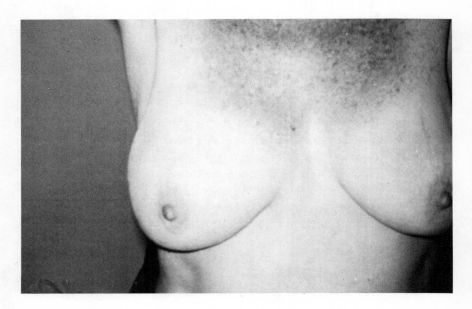

tissue that attach the breast to the chest wall and help maintain its upright position weaken, stretch, and permit the breast to sag.

The changes in the breast attributable to the aging process can be retarded somewhat by certain measures. First, women must avoid overweight as this will stretch the skin, weaken the fibrous bands that maintain the breast's position on the chest wall and cause it to sag. Since the skin at menopause has lost a good deal of its elastic resilience, it will not return to its previous appearance even after return to normal weight. Conversely, women who permit themselves to become too thin will discover that the skin overlying their breasts wrinkles and the organs sag.

Physical fitness is reflected in every organ of the body, including the breast. It is therefore important if one wants to hold on to a more youthful appearance, to exercise regularly. Such exercise will help maintain strength in the pectoral muscles and will help prevent stretching and weakening of the fibrous tissue fibers extending from the breast to the chest wall.

In some women, particularly those who are experiencing severe menopausal symptoms, the breasts become very tender to the touch and the nipples become extremely sensitive when caressed or kissed. The same type of reaction may occur when large doses of estrogen are administered repeatedly to relieve symptoms of menopause. The cause of this hypersensitivity is not understood, nor is there any form of satisfactory treatment to overcome the symptoms. Along with the tenderness and nipple sensitivity, there may be visible swelling of the breast and redness and enlargement of the nipple.

Many women today take estrogen regularly to relieve menopausal symptoms; others take it in the hope that it will retard signs of aging in their skin and will maintain the fullness of their breasts. On microscopic examination of tissue removed from the breast of a postmenopausal woman on large doses of estrogens, one frequently sees an extraordinary amount of active gland tissue. In other words, the breast microscopically looks like that of a much younger woman. But regardless of the limited extent estrogen may accomplish these goals, it must be kept in mind that these are powerful substances that should never be taken without the advice and supervision of a physician. Specifically, a woman with chronic cystic disease of the breasts (in which there can be hundreds of tiny cysts scattered throughout both breasts) or one who has had intraductal papillomatosis (the condition in which the cells lining the milk ducts are overgrown) should not take estrogens as it may activate these conditions. Nature intended the breast to become inactive after change of life, and it should be stimulated by hormones only if one can rest assured that the stimulation will not cause a dormant disease process to be reactivated.

Questions and Answers

Will the intermittent enlargement of the breasts prior to and accompanying menstruation continue after menopause if a woman is put on estrogen therapy?

Yes, if the estrogens are given cyclically. This means that the estrogens are given for a period of approximately three weeks and then discontinued for a week.

Should ovarian hormones be given to a woman in order to maintain the youthful appearance of her breasts?

Most gynecologists do not believe that this is a sufficient reason for hormone therapy. If, however, there are severe menopausal symptoms, they often will prescribe estrogen-containing hormones, and a side effect of their administration will be a fullness and more youthful appearance of the breasts.

Can plastic surgery on the breasts be successfully performed on women past menopause?

Yes. With the longer life-span and the increased desire of older women to retain their youthful appearance, plastic surgery on the breasts is being performed increasingly. Although vanity usually stimulates a woman's decision to undergo a plastic operation, there are frequently medical advantages. Older women with heavy pendulous breasts receive great relief through plastic surgery too.

Can reduction of an oversized breast be carried out successfully in women past menopause?

Yes.

Can augmentation of an undersized breast be carried out successfully in women past menopause?

Yes, but these procedures are much more successful when performed on younger patients.

How often should women past menopause have their breasts examined by a physician?

Twice each year. If this practice is adhered to, tumors can be discovered during the early stage. Four out of five cancers of the breast can be cured if they are discovered before they have spread to surrounding lymph glands.

Should women at menopause, or older, continue to practice self-examination of their breasts?

Yes. They should do it on the first day of each month if they have stopped having periods.

Do the breasts ever enlarge as one approaches menopause?

This occasionally does happen. It is thought to be due to an imbalance in ovarian hormone secretion that occurs during this time of life.

Do the nipples ever become unusually tender during the menopausal years?

Yes, in some women the tenderness is so great that there is discomfort even from wearing a brassiere.

What is the significance of a lump in the breast of a woman who has passed the menopause?

Unfortunately, many of the lumps that develop in the breasts of women past menopause are malignant. However, there are benign tumors, such as fatty tumors and areas of fat necrosis (degeneration), which develop after menopause. In addition, older women who lose a great deal of weight may discover in the breast a deep lump that has gone unnoticed for many years. Such lumps are almost always benign.

What causes painful breasts in women past menopause?

They occur in women who are markedly obese and whose breasts are pendulous. They also occur in older women who are receiving large doses of female sex hormones. Another cause is an inflammation within the breast (mastitis), occasionally appearing as a complication of a virus infection that has traveled throughout the body. Finally, pain in the breasts may sometimes be brought on by improperly fitting brassieres.

Does the tendency to form cysts subside after menopause?
Yes.

Will the giving of hormones to a menopausal woman cause cysts to form?
In some instances, yes. If a woman had a tendency toward cyst formation prior to menopause, as in cases of fibrocystic disease, the hormones may stimulate new cysts to form. However, I have never seen a case of breast cancer that could be attributed to the taking of estrogens.

What is the significance of a discharge from the nipple in a woman past menopause?
This usually indicates that there is a tumor within the ducts of the breast. In many such cases, the lump cannot be felt. Secretion from the nipple occasionally takes place with a patient who is under intensive hormone treatment.

What is the significance of a chronic ulcer or sore on the nipple?
This often indicates the presence of a malignant tumor in the breast. The appearance of such an ulcer should stimulate a woman to seek medical advice promptly.

Can a blow or injury to the breast cause cancer to develop?
No. Many women relate the onset of a breast tumor to a blow or injury they received. The explanation is as follows. Such a woman is unaware that she has a lump until she receives a blow on the breast. The pain occasioned by the blow causes her to examine the breast and she discovers a lump that has been there for some time.

Are malignant diseases of the breast more common in women who are far past the menopause than they are in younger menopausal women?
No. Statistics show that cancer of the breast occurs more often in women between the ages of forty-five and fifty years of age.

Is cancer of the breast in older women curable?

Yes. Malignant tumors tend to grow more slowly in older women, thus giving them a better chance for cure than many younger women. Of course, they must seek medical care early in the course of the disease.

Is it safe for women past the menopause to undergo extensive surgery for the removal of a breast cancer?

Yes. Even the most radical breast-removal operation can be tolerated by older women provided they are in a satisfactory state of general health. Only when someone is debilitated or has severe heart, liver, or kidney disease will extensive breast surgery be poorly tolerated.

Can older women tolerate X-ray or cobalt treatments for breast cancer?

Yes.

Are breast infections or abscesses common in women at or past menopause?

No. They are quite uncommon.

12 DISEASE PREVENTION AND EARLY DETECTION THROUGH BREAST EXAMINATION: BY SELF AND PHYSICIAN

Hundreds of millions of dollars are spent each year in America urging women to buy this or that hair shampoo or spray, or insisting on the need for various wonderful underarm deodorants and marvelous substances to improve "feminine hygiene." Yet only a trickle of money goes toward impressing upon them the essentiality of caring for their breasts!

It is shocking that so visible an organ of the body can be afflicted with undetected major disease for so long that it often reaches an incurable stage. The explanation for this situation is not simple. Most women *are* aware that they should undergo periodic medical examinations and they know, too, that a lump in the breast is rather readily diagnosed. One must conclude, therefore, that women refrain from self-examination or examination by a doctor because they are so fearful that something wrong *will* be discovered. If this theory is correct, these fears must be overcome before women will submit to regular breast examination.

Curiously, great strides have been made in convincing women to seek periodic pelvic examinations and Pap smears. It would seem that the female psyche is better able to adjust to the possible surgical loss of the uterus than it is to the loss of a mammary gland. If so, such reluctance is understandable since the former procedure is unaccompanied by outward disfigurement.

To set the record straight and to allay fear, *the overwhelming majority of abnormal findings in a breast are not cancerous.* Well over 90 percent of all breast lumps fall into this category. And more than 90 percent of cancers of the breast can be cured if they are discovered early, before they have reached a centimeter or two in diameter (2½ centimeters to the inch), or have spread to neighboring lymph nodes or to distant parts of the body. Early detection is the key to breast cancer's curability.

All women who are still having periods should examine their breasts on the day menstruation ends. Postmenopausal women should conduct breast self-examination on the first day of each month. Women between twenty-five and thirty-five years of age, in addition to seeking physician examination whenever a lump is felt or whenever there are any symptoms relative to the breasts, should have a yearly checkup by their physician. Women over thirty-five years of age should undergo a semiannual breast examination by a doctor.

Breast self-examination, however, must not be used as a substitute for an examination by a physician. One cannot become so expert in self-examination that one can assume the sole responsibility in diagnosing the presence or absence of a tumor within the organ. The great advantage of self-examination is that most women can detect some difference in the feel of their breasts when the examination is conducted on a month-to-month basis. These changes may be obscured if a woman indulges in too frequent self-examination. For this reason, unless a lump is felt accidentally at some other time, self-examination should be conducted only once a month.

Patients often ask what sort of doctor should conduct their periodic breast examination. In response to this question, one might analogize by saying that the gynecologist is best trained to examine the pelvic organs, the dermatologist the skin, and the ophthalmologist the eyes. The surgeon is best trained in examination of the breast. Of course, if a patient is undergoing a general physical examination by her family physician, he will examine the breasts and will undoubtedly recommend further examination by a surgeon if he uncovers a lump.

There is a great advantage, if one is satisfied with the care she has been receiving, in having the same doctor carry out the periodic breast examinations. If an area of possible disease has been felt in a breast on one occasion, the physician will make note of it on the patient's chart and may also make a sketch of the breast denoting the exact location of the area in question. Then, when the patient returns some time later, the physician will be able to compare present findings with those of the previous examination. He may also recommend mammography, that is, an X ray of the breast, at the time of each examination and will be able to compare the two sets of pictures to see if there have been changes. However, it is seldom that changes will be seen on mammograms unless an interval of several weeks or months has elapsed.

Women must train themselves not to be too upset on being told that a particular spot in the breast requires observation. As we have mentioned elsewhere, the breast is an extremely active organ, subject to wide fluctuations in its function due to the secretions of the hormones circulating in the blood. As a consequence, a thickened area or palpable lump may be present on one examination but not on another. Also, a lump may become smaller rather than larger within a few days' or weeks' time. For these reasons, it is not at all unusual for the examining physician to suggest a return visit for reexamination. In this connection, most experts in breast disease prefer to examine a breast containing a doubtful mass during the intermenstrual period when the organ is quiescent and free from the engorgement brought on by approaching menstruation.

Examination of the breasts by a physician is a very simple, painless procedure, differing relatively little from that employed in self-examination. In addition, he will examine the axillary (underarm) region to note whether the lymph nodes are enlarged, and he may explore the area just above the collarbone. In addition, he may transilluminate or shine a light through the breast to see if any abnormal shadows are present. Finally, he may recommend that the patient undergo mammography and, in rare instances, thermography, a diagnostic technique based on heat radiation.

Self-examination, to be meaningful, must be conducted with the correct technique. It is not at all difficult to perform and can be taught to any patient by her physician within a few minutes' time. In brief, this is how it should be done:

1. Lie flat in bed face up. Place a small pillow or large telephone directory under the right shoulder and back of your chest. This prevents the breast from sagging to the side of the body, thus permitting a more satisfactory examination.

2. Place your right arm on top of your head.

3. Place the fingers of your left hand together in a straight position, and gently draw the flat portion of the fingers, not the tips, over the inner half of the breast, starting at the top and working down toward the bottom of the breast. It is easier for some women to feel a lump if their fingers are moistened with a little mineral or baby oil, or soap. This allows the fingers to glide smoothly over the breast.

4. Lower your right arm and place it at your side.

5. Again, take the flat portion of the fingers of your left hand and glide them over the outer half of the breast toward the nipple. Start this at the top of the breast and work down toward the bottom of the breast.

6. Repeat the above maneuvers, in reverse, for examination of the left breast.

7. Milk each nipple gently but firmly to note any discharge. Normally, there is no discharge.

8. After completing the above, stand in front of a mirror in a good light and inspect your breasts. Look particularly for the following abnormalities:

> a. A sore or ulceration of the nipple.
> b. A change in the size of a breast.
> c. A change in the level of one of the nipples.
> d. A change in the appearance of the skin overlying the breast, especially a dimpling or indentation in its contours.
> e. The presence of a lump or a protrusion of any part of the breast.

Most lumps are sufficiently superficial so that they can be felt by the gentle gliding of the fingers over the breast surface. In doing this, it is

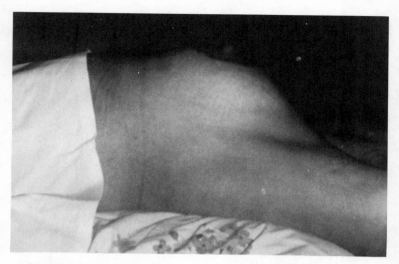

Self-examination: Woman lies flat in bed with a small pillow under her shoulder and upper chest region. Left breast is shown here.

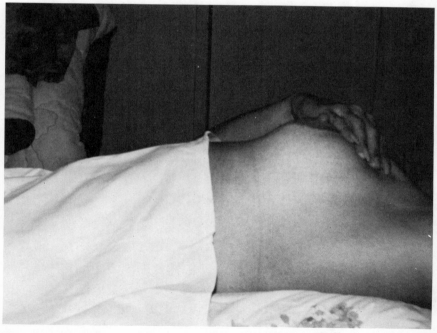

The right hand, with fingers extended, is drawn slowly from left to right as it examines the upper outer portion of the left breast.

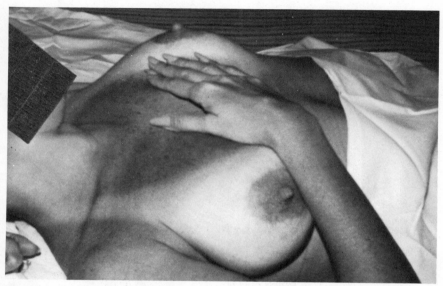

The right hand examines the upper inner portion of the left breast as it continues to move to the right.

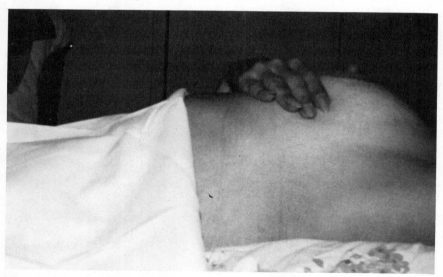

The right hand repeats the maneuver while examining the lower outer portion of the breast . . .

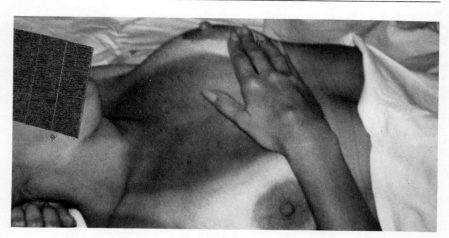

. . . and the lower inner portion of the breast. The pillow will then be placed under the right side of the shoulder and chest, and the left hand used to examine the right breast.

important that the examination be carried out with the *flat of the fingers* of the two distal joint regions. If the tips of the fingers are used, many lumps will be overlooked. Also, the fingers must not press hard into the breast as that, too, will obscure the ability to feel a lump. And finally, the breast should never be examined by squeezing a portion of it between the thumb and other fingers.

It has been argued that self-examination will ultimately result in unnecessary neurotic reactions among women. Whereas there is some truth to this belief, one must weigh this untoward possibility against the benefits accruing from the earlier detection of breast disease. Moreover, neurotic tendencies seldom arise because of a particular practice. A neurotic may become slightly more neurotic through self-examination, but a well-adjusted individual will not abruptly turn into a neurotic simply because she examines her breasts once a month. Every once in a while a physician encounters a patient who is so apprehensive about breast cancer that she examines herself every few days. These women should be advised not to engage in self-examination at all. Instead, they should be examined by their doctor every other month. If they follow this routine they can be safely assured that a tumor, developed during the interval since the previous examination, will not grow to proportions beyond control.

Questions and Answers

Is self-examination of the breasts advisable?
Yes.

Should self-examination be used instead of examination by a physician?
No. It should be only a supplement to regular examination by a doctor.

How often should a woman examine her breasts?
Once each month.

Is self-examination always accurate?
Not always, but it is frequently helpful in discovering a lump that might otherwise be overlooked.

At what time of the month should a woman examine her breasts?
If she is still having periods, she should conduct self-examination the day the period ends. If she is postmenopausal, she should examine her breasts on the first day of each month.

Can a husband be trained to examine his wife's breasts?
Yes, but curiously, a husband is more apt to miss a lump than the woman.

Can the breasts be harmed by too strenuous self-examination?
No.

How soon after a woman finds a lump in her breast should she go for medical examination?
Within a few days.

Do some lumps in the breast disappear spontaneously?
Yes, but these are usually not true lumps. More often they represent swelling of the breast associated with menstruation or a hormone imbalance.

Is it more difficult for a woman with nodular breasts or cystic disease of the breasts to conduct a meaningful examination?

Yes. In some cases the general lumpiness is so marked that self-examination is not advisable.

Should a pregnant woman practice self-examination?

Usually not. Breast engorgement during pregnancy will make it too difficult for her to feel a lump.

Can a nursing mother conduct a meaningful self-examination?

Usually not. The general engorgement of the breast during the nursing period will make it too difficult for her to feel a lump.

Is mammography a substitute for self-examination of the breasts?

No. Mammography frequently does not reveal a lump that a woman can feel through self-examination.

Should the average woman undergo periodic mammography?

Women over 35 years of age should undergo mammography once a year.

How accurate is examination by a physician in determining the presence or absence of a lump in the breast?

Very accurate if the examining physician is familiar with breast disease.

Can a physician usually distinguish between a benign lump and a malignant one merely by examination of the breasts?

In many cases, he can; in others this distinction can be made only after removing the suspicious lump and submitting it for microscopic examination.

How often should a woman with known cystic disease go for breast examination?

At least three times a year.

How often should a woman who has had a benign cyst or tumor removed surgically go for follow-up breast examination?
At least three times a year.

How frequently should a woman who has had a breast removed for cancer go for follow-up examination?
Three times a year.

13 BREAST INJURIES

All people are endowed with automatic reflexes that protect their bodies from harm. The eyelids blink automatically when a blow is imminent; the hand pulls away the instant it touches something hot; the pelvis contracts to avert an injury to the genital area. Instinctual reactions protect the breasts, and physicians who treat large numbers of accident cases are frequently amazed how often these exposed and unprotected structures escape trauma. It is not at all unusual to see a woman who has sustained severe multiple injuries to her head, neck, shoulders, and arms, yet suffers no damage to her breasts. If one had a slow-motion picture of such an accident in progress, he would see that the shoulders, arms, and hands tend to move to cover and protect the breasts. In other words, most breast injuries result from accidents in which there has been no warning.

The breast contains a good blood supply with many small, fragile veins and arteries. It is also composed of a great deal of fat. As a consequence, blows to the breast generally result in hemorrhage and destruction of fat cells. A lump usually forms within minutes or hours following a striking blow as blood seeps into the breast substance. The area swells and becomes increasingly tender to the touch.

Most direct injuries to the breast subside spontaneously over a period of several days, although the lump created by the trauma may persist for several weeks. Ordinarily, the blood clot that has collected at the site of the injury will be absorbed, as will the injured fat cells. Mention has not been made of damage to the milk ducts or secreting glands as these structures are seldom involved in the average breast injury. Of course, a bullet or stab wound or a laceration may involve these tissues, but these are infrequent occurrences.

In especially severe traumas, the hemorrhage may result in a hematoma, a localized collection of blood. The hematoma can progress in one of three ways:

1. The blood clots and forms a hard lump that persists for several weeks.

2. The blood may become fluid and surrounded by a capsule. This is known as a hematocele.

3. The hematoma may absorb rapidly within a few days' time.

No treatment is necessary for a hematoma that is obviously absorbing. One will know this by the fact that the lump gets progressively smaller. A hematoma that fluidifies may require a surgical incision to let out the blood. Following this procedure, the lump disappears quickly.

Damaged fat tissue may absorb completely, or may undergo slow necrosis, with the formation of a permanent, hard lump. Such a lump is occasionally diagnosed erroneously as a cancer. However, breast injuries do *not* cause cancer.

But in some instances a woman's attention is first called to a tumor in her breast by an injury in the vicinity of a preexisting lump. One of my patients was struck in the breast by a golf ball. A lump formed in the area and failed to absorb over a period of two months. Surgery was undertaken in anticipation of cleaning out a large hematoma, but when the breast was incised, a large malignant tumor was found adjacent to the site struck by the golf ball. Had the injury not taken place, the malignancy might have gone undetected indefinitely. More frequently, a converse situation is encountered: When surgery is carried out with a preoperative diagnosis of cancer, a hematoma or area of fat necrosis is encountered. Women sometimes forget an injury that has occurred long previously. I operated on a woman whose breast felt as if it contained a tumor, and whose mammogram strongly indicated possible cancer. She gave no history of a breast injury but, at surgery, I found an old blood clot. Postoperatively, on refreshing her memory, she recalled that several months previously, a co-worker had accidentally struck her breast with her elbow. The pain had not been great and the patient had forgotten the incident.

Any lump secondary to an injury should be watched carefully so that it is not misinterpreted. A lump that fails to disappear within a month's time should, in all probability, be biopsied. Only in this way can one be absolutely certain that the lump does not, in fact, represent a preexisting tumor.

Breast injuries already mentioned include those from excessively ardent or sadistic lovers—a high incidence. Nipple biting can cause a serious breast infection, causing abscess formation or cellulitis (inflammation of the connective tissues). Undue pinching or squeezing may cause hemorrhage into the tissues with a resultant hematoma. Here, too, these injuries do not lead to cancer.

Another frequent cause of breast injury is burn. Women who cook should be particularly careful not to wear flammable negligees or garments that can easily catch fire. Flowing collars and sleeves all too often make contact with an open gas range or oven and ignite, producing serious burns about the breasts. And breast burns occur from the spilling of hot liquids. Also, women should be very careful with faucets while in a shower; the showerhead generally points directly at the chest region, and if someone unthinkingly turns the wrong faucet, on or off, a severe scald can result.

Burns of the breast area are extremely painful and may take weeks to heal. Conscious caution in the kitchen and in the shower are the best preventives.

With the increased physical activity of modern women, along with the advanced speed and mechanization of society, we can expect a greater potential for accidents—and breast injuries. We might counter this with a greater awareness, if not with a good supporting brassiere.

Questions and Answers

How long does it take the average lump due to an injury to disappear?
Within two to three weeks. If it persists after that time, either a hematoma has formed or destruction of fat tissue has set in.

What is fat necrosis?
It is destruction of fat tissue. The end result may be the formation of a hard, irregular lump.

Does fat destruction ever take place in a woman who sustains repeated pressure on the breast while at work?

Yes. Some women lean against machines while at work. If they continue this practice over a period of years, it can lead to areas of localized fat necrosis.

Is it sometimes difficult to distinguish an area of fat necrosis from a breast cancer?

Yes.

What is the treatment for a lump thought to be caused by fat destruction within the breast?

It should be biopsied to make certain no cancer exists.

Does inflammation of the veins of the breast ever result from injury?

Yes, phlebitis of the veins of the breast may result from local injury.

How can one make a diagnosis of phlebitis of the breast?

One will see a streak of bluish discoloration following the course of the veins that lead from the nipple up toward the armpit. On feeling the area there is a cordlike, firm sensation along the course of the vein.

Does phlebitis of the breast cause pain?

In its early stages the inflamed vein may be quite tender.

Do most cases of phlebitis subside without any harmful aftereffects?

Yes, within a few weeks' time. No treatment is necessary.

Do women frequently attribute a lump to an injury rather than to a tumor?

Yes. Since most women at one time or another sustain some kind of injury, they are quick to attribute a lump to such injury. It is, of course, a happier diagnosis than that of a tumor.

Can one often distinguish between a lump in the breast that has been caused by an injury and one that is due to a tumor?

Yes. Most injuries subside within a few weeks' time, leaving no lump behind. However, the distinction cannot always be made, and for this reason, a biopsy is frequently advised when a lump is persistent.

Can a mammogram distinguish between a lump caused by an injury and one caused by a tumor?
Yes, in some cases. However, the surgeon's opinion is more valuable than a mammographic finding. When doubt exists, a biopsy should be performed.

Do hematomas of the breast ever form fluid and give the appearance of being a cyst?
Yes.

Does breast injury frequently follow the nursing of a child?
No. However, some infants with teeth do bite the nipple, especially when they can't get enough milk.

Does an injury to the breast often cause discharge from the nipple?
No. Duct injuries are uncommon.

14 BREAST INFECTIONS

Since the breast is covered most of the time and is therefore out of contact with dirt and bacteria-laden substances, it avoids many of the infections that afflict exposed parts of the body. The main circumstances surrounding breast infection are:

1. Nursing.
2. Biting of the nipple during nursing or lovemaking.
3. Blockage of one of the main ducts of the breast.
4. Involvement secondary to a disease affecting other organs of the body.
5. Infection secondary to an infected sebaceous cyst, pimple, or boil.
6. Abscess in a newborn infant, associated with milk secretion.

1. The nursing breast has repeated contact with the bacteria within the mouth of the infant. These bacteria are present normally in every newborn from the very first day of life. At any time during the period of breast-feeding, a slight abrasion or crack in the nipple may occur and bacteria enter the breast through these areas. Inasmuch as many women have decreased resistance to bacterial infection during the few weeks after childbirth, their tissues may not be able to overcome the bacterial invasion. The breast becomes red, hot, swollen, and tender about the nipple, and the inflammation may spread to the deeper tissues.

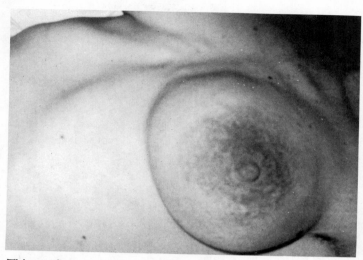

This mother was able to overcome her breast infection without discontinuing her nursing. Antibiotics and warm soaks controlled the infection seen here.

Mastitis of lactation, as infection in the nursing breast is called, may subside spontaneously within a few days or may proceed to abscess formation. Treatment consists of administration of large doses of antibiotics, specifically those that are effective against the staphylococcus, streptococcus, and E. coli germs. If it appears that the breast infection is being controlled with the antibiotics, plus the use of warm compresses, nursing may be continued. If, on the other hand, it is obvious that an abscess has formed requiring surgical incision and drainage, then nursing must be discontinued. The infant suffers no harm from nursing at an inflamed, or even infected, breast.

2. A bite of the nipple may produce an abrasion or actual laceration. Occasionally, such a bite inadvertently takes place as a mother is nursing an older infant who already has cut a tooth. More often, the nipple injury is secondary to suckling or biting during the foreplay of lovemaking. As described above, bacteria enter the deeper tissues of the breast through these abrasions or lacerations. Again, the medical treatment of the breast infection will consist of warm, wet compresses and the administration of

antibiotic drugs. If the infection progresses to abscess formation, incision and drainage are indicated.

3. The major ducts of the breast come together beneath the nipple. In rare instances, a papilloma, or warty growth, within a duct grows and obstructs the passageway. Most of these papillomas secrete small amounts of liquid (serum) that dam up in the duct behind the growth. The stagnant serum tends to become infected and may produce an inflammation of the duct and surrounding breast tissue. Or, in some cases, an infection from the duct may burrow through the breast tissue beneath the nipple and gain exit through the skin. When this happens, a duct fistula has formed. Surgical excision of the fistula is necessary, or a discharge from the breast will continue to take place intermittently for an indefinite period of time.

4. Any systemic infection, such as tuberculosis, syphilis, actinomycosis, anthrax, and so on, may spread from its site of origin to other parts of the body. Thus, the breast may become infected from a distant source. Except in impoverished and deprived sections of the world, tuberculosis is pretty well controlled by the prompt administration of one or more of the excellent antituberculosis drugs. As a consequence, breast involvement in this disease is rarely encountered in this country.

Syphilis, too, usually receives early treatment and is arrested before it reaches its tertiary stage. However, in neglected cases, a syphilitic abscess, known as a gumma, may attack the breast. This is a late complication of the disease, not appearing until many years after the initial infection.

In all secondary breast infections, cure relies on the adequate treatment of the general systemic disease.

5. Pimples, boils, and infected sebaceous cysts may be located in the skin of the breast, as they may appear anywhere on the body's surface. Infection of underlying breast tissue seldom ensues unless the individual squeezes the infected area, thus spreading bacteria. If these infections come to a head, they should be opened surgically.

6. Newborn infants whose breasts secrete milk are particularly prone to abscess formation. This results because the tiny ducts become obstructed and the milk secretions dam up under the nipple. The infection clears rapidly following simple incision and drainage.

Questions and Answers

Are breast infections common?

No, but like all structures in the body, the breasts are susceptible to bacterial invasion.

Are breast abscesses easily diagnosed?

Not always. An abscess deep within the breast may never point toward the surface, thus making diagnosis difficult.

Do breast infections ever cause swelling of the glands in the armpit?

Yes, since the lymphatic channels from the breast lead to the lymph nodes (glands) in the armpit. These glands may become markedly enlarged and tender.

Do breast infections often travel to distant parts of the body?

No. It is rare for this to occur.

Do breast abscesses ever appear as multiple lesions affecting various areas of breast substance?

Yes, especially if the infection has been neglected or goes untreated for a long period of time.

Are breast infections a frequent accompaniment of nursing?

This is probably the most common cause of breast infection. However, the overall incidence of breast infection secondary to nursing is not great.

Should a mother continue to nurse despite the fact that she has an inflamed breast?

Yes, in some instances. But when a true abscess has formed and has been drained surgically, an open wound results. Under such circumstances, nursing must be discontinued.

Do infections of the breast tend to become chronic?

Not unless they have gone untreated.

What is mastitis?

The term means "inflammation of the breast." However, the term *chronic cystic mastitis* has been abandoned as it is now known that no bacterial or viral invasion is associated with the condition.

What is inflammatory cancer of the breast?

It is a rare form of cancer occurring during pregnancy. There is no real inflammation accompanying the tumor; it derives its name from the fact that the breast appears red and feels hot when this type of cancer is present.

Is inflammatory cancer of the breast caused by a bacterium?
No.

Does a breast infection make one prone to develop cancer?
No.

15 BREAST PAIN

Every woman at one time or another experiences some breast pain. If it occurs at widely separated intervals and lasts but a short time, most women ignore it. When the pain persists for several hours or days, or when it recurs frequently, it creates considerable apprehension. The concern may initiate self-examination to discover if a lump is present, and if any doubt exists, the woman usually rushes to see her physician.

Painful breasts, known as mammalgia, or isolated instances of pain, may originate from any one of several sources. The most common reasons for breast pain are:

1. Cyclic or periodic pain. This type comes on during the two or three days immediately preceding the onset of menstruation. Although cyclic pain may be located anywhere within the breast, it is likely to be most marked in the outer and upper outer regions. Along with the pain, it is customary to experience considerable tenderness to the touch. This is the pain in the breast thought to be due to the increased blood supply and consequent swelling that prevails at this time of the month, discussed earlier. It is not considered to be associated with a true disease process. The pain and the tenderness disappear by the end of the second or third day of menstruation.

Some women complain so bitterly of premenstrual breast pain that it handicaps their activity greatly. Study of the makeup of these individuals often reveals that they are emotionally disturbed and overreact to other stressful situations, too.

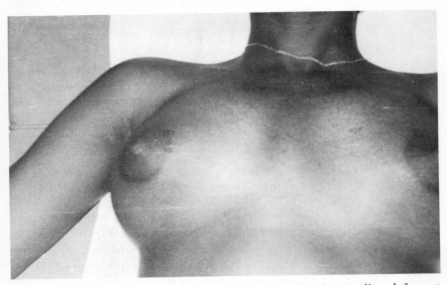

Full-breasted women with gland tissue high up on the chest wall and far out toward the underarm area are most likely to suffer recurrent breast pain.

2. Axillary breast tissue. The normal extension of breast tissue up toward the armpit is known as the tail of the breast. In some women, mainly those with large breasts, the amount of breast tissue in the axilla, or underarm area, is greater than normal. This tissue will be involved in the swelling and engorgement that takes place each month with the onset of menstruation and will cause an aggravation of symptoms in those women who normally suffer periodic pain. The edge of the brassiere frequently presses upon this already painful area, causing even greater aggravation of symptoms. Occasionally, in order to relieve this condition, surgical removal of the tail of the breast is indicated. A small incision approximately two inches long is made in the upper outer portion of the breast and the entire tail is removed. The operative procedure is simple, recovery is complete within a few days, and relief of symptoms is striking.

3. An extremely common cause of painful breasts is the wearing of an improperly fitting brassiere. Such pain is encountered in women with very large, pendulous breasts who wear too large bras with too little uplift, and in women who try to camouflage the amplitude of their busts by wearing too tight brassieres.

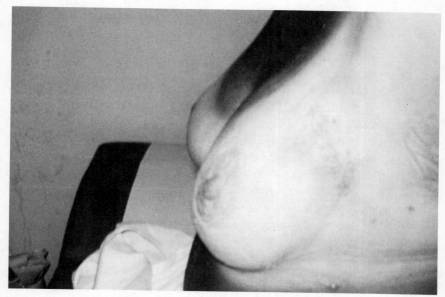

This scar near the armpit results from removing the tail of the breast. The patient's continual pain was completely relieved following this operation. The scar will fade.

Some physicians think that the pain felt by those with unusually large, pendulous breasts is the result of a stretching of the fibrous connective tissues that attach the breast to the underlying chest wall. A characteristic sign in these patients is exquisite tenderness on finger pressure on the chest wall just above the breast in the region of the third rib.

4. Breast pain of emotional origin can be diagnosed readily by the fact that it follows no definite functional or disease pattern. It may appear premenstrually or at any other time of the month; it may localize to the outer portions of the breast or to any other part; it may be dull, sharp, or burning in character; it may be fleeting or may last for hours or days.

Investigation of the patient's personality and character may reveal unusual neurotic components. In my experience, many of the women who complain of a continually painful breast show no breast pathology, seem to have poor marriages, sexual hangups, and an excessive fear of cancer. Assurance that nothing is wrong with their breast does not always dispel the pain because the underlying emotional instability has not been eliminated. However, the best one can do for these women is to let them visit their physician whenever they wish and to reassure them each time that no breast pathology is present. The worst one can do is treat them with hormones or tranquilizers for this will convince them that their breast pain is organic rather than psychic in origin.

Some women with painful breasts attribute their symptoms to activities incurred during sexual intercourse. Whereas the breasts may be somewhat turgid and sore as the result of strenuous manipulation and suckling prior to and during intercourse, such pain lasts but a brief time and ordinarily causes little concern. These patients should be assured that permanent harm does not result from breast participation in a normal sexual contact, nor will a cancer eventuate.

Of course, there are exceptions when a sadistic male bites and pinches the breast so strenuously that he produces a real trauma.

5. Pain secondary to trauma—intense squeezing, pinching, or biting during so-called love play; more often, a direct blow from contact with a protruding object or by a fist. Also, in chapter 7 it was pointed out that the metal stays of a poorly fitting bra may create breast pain as can a brassiere that is too tight.

6. Pain secondary to infection, characterized by swelling, heat, redness, and tenderness. The pain is continuous and is not relieved until the infection subsides spontaneously or pus is drained surgically from the infected area.

7. Most isolated cysts of the breast are painless but once in a while a cyst grows to large proportions within a few days. When this happens, the cyst may cause considerable pain in the area. Also, hemorrhage into a cyst occasionally takes place, and when it does, pain usually results.

Cystic disease of the breasts sometimes causes pain before and during menstruation. This is akin to cyclic pain, described above.

8. Breast tumors seldom cause pain although many women do attribute pain to the area of a lump. Such pain in most cases is psychological in origin. Extensive studies on this subject reveal that pain is not a constant symptom of breast cancer, being present in less than 1 of 20 women with the disease. When it does occur, it is usually the result of pressure on the tumor by contact with a hard object.

9. Postoperative pain secondary to the local removal of a cyst or tumor is not very intense. It is surprising how little pain follows even a

large incision or one that surrounds part of the nipple. Most patients require a minimum of pain-relieving drugs for the first or second postoperative day, and none thereafter.

There is considerable pain secondary to breast removal (mastectomy). It is usually located in the chest wall, in the front and back of the shoulder, and in the arm. The pain is caused by the necessity of disturbing nerves originating from the brachial plexus, the bundle of nerves coursing from the neck to the arm. Many patients suffer from this aching pain for weeks or months, occasionally longer, after a mastectomy.

10. Pain secondary to cracked nipples or caked breasts. A mother with cracked nipples may be in such pain when nursing that she is forced to wean her baby. Proper care of the breast during pregnancy can often prevent this unpleasant condition.

Caked breasts secondary to retained milk is an extremely uncomfortable condition associated with marked pain and tenderness. Today, due to the prompt administration of Deladumone or stilbestrol for a woman who decides not to breast-feed her child, caked breasts seldom ensue.

11. Pain of undetermined origin. There are women who suffer occasional transient breast pain who fall into none of the categories discussed above. They are not neurotic nor do they have inordinate cancerophobia. The pain may be sharp or dull, it may be transient or continue for several hours, and center on the nipple or elsewhere in the breast.

The explanation for this type of pain is not really known, except that fleeting pain occasionally afflicts any part of the body without real disease being present. People sometimes have a transient backache, pain in a joint, a muscle ache, a headache, and so on. In all probability there is a temporary irritation of nerve endings that transmit the sensation of pain from the periphery to the brain. The breast, being a rather sizable organ, is richly supplied with nerves and one might therefore expect it, too, to be the site of pain sensations.

Suffice it to say that transient breast pain is unimportant and requires no treatment.

Questions and Answers

Do most women at one or another time have pain in their breasts?
Yes.

Is most pain in the breast constant or intermittent?

Intermittent, unless it has been caused by an injury, and infection, or a hemorrhage into a cyst.

Are painful breasts, unassociated with a lump, usually tender to the touch?

No.

How often should a woman go for an examination if she regularly suffers pain in the breast?

No more than the patient without pain. Women under 35 years of age should have a breast examination at least once a year; those over 35, twice a year.

When is pain felt by a patient with a solid benign tumor?

When an injury is inflicted in the region of the tumor.

Should a woman take hormones to overcome painful breasts?

Only if there is a definite hormone imbalance. It is possible that the administration of hormones, when not specifically indicated, will cause more imbalance and will fail to overcome the breast pain.

Should a woman take diuretic drugs to overcome the pain seen just prior to menstruation?

Some women are relieved by this medication, but it should be taken only when prescribed by a physician.

Should a woman who is subject to painful breasts refrain from having her breasts caressed and kissed during intercourse?

No, but her mate should know that gentleness is essential to prevent pain after lovemaking.

What is the significance of a burning sensation in the breasts?

Usually, it has no medical significance.

Should a woman ignore a lump in the breasts just because it is painless?

No. Most breast tumors are painless.

16 BIOPSY AND CYTOLOGY

Biopsy is the removal of tissues from the body and the submission of them for gross and microscopic examination by a pathologist. Cytology means the examination of cells from the body for the same purpose. The pathologist is the medical specialist who is expert in diagnosing disease processes through gross and microscopic examination of cells or tissues.

The breast surgeon should and does work closely with the pathologist and, no matter how expert he may be in clinical diagnosis when he examines a lump that he has removed, he never decides on a final course of action until his diagnosis has been confirmed by pathological examination. In this way, the patient has double the protection she would have if the decision to proceed depended solely on the surgeon's examination of the excised specimen.

It is standard practice in all accredited hospitals in this country for patients with surgical breast disease to undergo biopsy, prior to, during, or after surgery. After the biopsy report has been received, and it is positive, the surgeon will proceed to perform the operation indicated by the diagnosis. If a positive, conclusive diagnosis is not apparent even with the help of the gross and microscopic examination by the pathologist, the surgeon will close the operative wound, return his patient to the recovery room, and wait as long as is necessary—perhaps for several days—until a precise diagnosis of the lesion has been reached. It has been found in

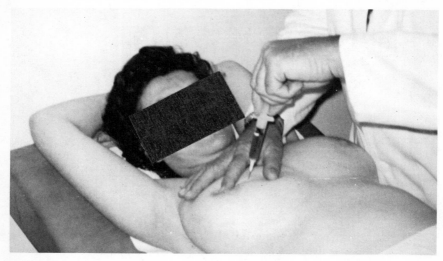

The fluid removed from this breast cyst will be sent to the laboratory for cytological examination for cancer cells.

several excellent studies conducted at various cancer institutions that ultimate survival or cure in breast cancer is not influenced by the few days' interval between the initial surgery for biopsy purposes and the definitive operation for eradication of the lesion.

Exact diagnosis of the submitted material is possible in about 98 to 99 percent of cases when interpretation is made by a pathologist who is expert in the field of breast pathology. This, of course, means that one or two patients out of every hundred must endure the stress of waiting out the period until an absolute diagnosis can be made. For this reason, it is important that women be told before initial surgery that every once in a while a patient must undergo this unpleasant experience. They should also be informed that the delay does not necessarily mean that cancer will be the eventual diagnosis. On the contrary, in the majority of cases in which the pathologist is unable to reach a diagnosis while the patient is under anesthesia, the ultimate diagnosis is that of a benign condition. (I recently operated on a woman who had had two previous operations for a benign breast lesion. The pathologists at the hospital, and at three other hospitals in the area, examined the microscopic slides of the tissue removed at surgery. Four thought the lesion to be benign; three judged it to be malignant; all agreed that the breast should not be removed but that the patient should be examined every two to three months to note whether the lesion grew back again.)

There are several types of cytological and biopsy examinations. These are:

1. Examination of fluid that exudes from the nipple. Microscopic studies of nipple discharges may reveal the presence of malignant cells. However, a negative biopsy does not necessarily mean that the underlying lesion is benign. Discharges may be negative for cancer cells even though the condition causing the discharge is malignant.

2. Examination of fluid withdrawn by needle and syringe from a cyst. Occasionally, a malignant growth is associated with a cyst, and examination of the fluid will reveal malignant cells.

3. Needle biopsy. This procedure, often performed in the surgeon's office under local anesthesia, is carried out by inserting a special biopsy needle into a growth and removing a tiny amount of tissue. This type of biopsy can also be done merely by inserting a large ordinary needle, attached to a syringe, into a lump and suctioning out a few cells. The cells are then spread on to a glass slide, stained, and examined under the microscope.

A positive needle biopsy is conclusive if it shows malignant cells. With this knowledge, the surgeon can proceed to perform definitive surgery for the cancer without further diagnostic procedures. However, a negative biopsy is not conclusive proof that the lesion is benign. It is entirely possible that the biopsy needle failed to enter the cancer-bearing portion of the lump or, even if it did, an insufficient number of cells were obtained to enable a diagnosis. *In other words, a positive needle biopsy obviates the need for further biopsy during surgery; a negative biopsy means that further examination must be carried out during surgery.*

Many surgeons prefer not to do needle biopsies in their offices because they are not as accurate as those carried out at the operating table. Moreover, if a patient learns from a needle biopsy done in a doctor's office that she has a malignancy, she is faced with the strain of waiting for a hospital bed to become available. In some areas, this interval may be as long as two to three weeks.

4. Incisional biopsy involves taking a piece of the tumor and submitting it for gross and microscopic examination during surgery. This type of biopsy is reserved for those patients with exceptionally large tumors, as ordinarily, it is just as simple to remove the entire lump as it is to excise a part of it.

5. Excisional biopsy is the procedure of choice. It is performed while the patient is under anesthesia. This involves removal of the entire lump and its submission to the pathologist for immediate gross and microscopic examination. The technique employed in preparing the specimen is known as frozen section. It involves quick-freezing the specimen, cutting it into very thin slices, staining it, and examining it under a microscope.

Today, frozen section biopsies are conducted in all accredited hospitals, and surgeons invariably await the pathologist's report before removing a patient's breast. As mentioned previously, neither excisional nor incisional biopsy is necessary if a positive needle biopsy has been obtained prior to surgery.

When the slightest doubt exists as to the diagnosis, the pathologist will urge the surgeon to close the wound and to wait until paraffin block sections can be made in the laboratory. This will allow the pathologist to cut many sections from different parts of the tumor and to study them at his leisure. This procedure takes two to three days, during which time the patient remains in the hospital.

Questions and Answers

How much tissue is removed in a biopsy?

A portion, or more often the entire lesion, is removed. The tissue is then submitted to a pathologist for gross and microscopic examination and diagnosis.

How long does it take a surgeon to perform a biopsy of a breast lump?
1. A needle biopsy requires 4 or 5 minutes to perform.
2. An incisional biopsy may take 15 to 20 minutes to perform.
3. An excisional biopsy may take 15 to 30 minutes to perform. Examination of the tissue by the pathologist requires an additional 15 to 30 minutes.

Is needle biopsy painful?

No. The surgeon will often inject a few drops of local anesthetic into the skin overlying the lump and this will eliminate pain.

When is incisional biopsy preferable to excisional biopsy?

When the lump in the breast is exceptionally large and it will take too long to do a total local removal of the mass.

How long an incision is made to perform a biopsy of a breast lesion?
Approximately 2 to 3 inches.

How long a hospital stay is necessary to carry out a biopsy of the breast?
Approximately 2 to 3 days.

17 MAMMOGRAPHY

Mammography is an X-ray technique especially devised for examination of the breasts. It is now advocated as a routine procedure to be performed each year in much the same manner as a Pap smear is recommended to uncover pathology of the genital organs.

Extensive studies have been carried out in this country on women who have been chosen at random from a large group of insured persons. In all instances, their breasts were found to be free of lumps on clinical examination by a physician. The studies involved approximately 32,500 women, but breast cancers were detected through mammography in 27 of them. If we now enlarge this sample so as to include the entire adult female population of the United States, one notes that *approximately 50,000 women are walking around with cancer of the breast even though there is no mass that can be felt by their doctors!*

According to statistics of the American Cancer Society, approximately 90,000 new cases of breast cancer appear each year, but one wonders how much greater this figure would be if all women actually did undergo a yearly mammography. And one wonders why, to date, women have failed to show the same interest in mammography as they have in Pap smear examinations.

Experts in mammography have found that the examination is at its most accurate when applied to older women because their breasts contain less glandular tissue and more fat. A deviation from normal can be spotted more readily on studying their X-ray films. It has also been noted that large breasts lend themselves more readily than small breasts to accurate interpretation.

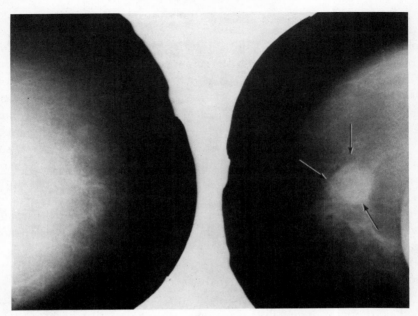

Mammography is a great aid to diagnosis when it shows a lesion suspicious of cancer. The mammogram on the left shows a normal breast. The one on the right shows a large cancer (*arrows*).

Recently, a newer version of mammographic technique has been developed that gives promise of even greater accuracy in diagnosing tumors during their very earliest stages. The technique is known as xeroradiography or xerography. It employs a selenium plate to take the X rays rather than the usual X-ray film. The method provides images of breast structure with a very high degree of contrast. Also, xerography requires less than half the amount of X-ray exposure that the conventional mammograph uses.

One of the difficulties in mammography, especially in xeroradiography, is that not all X-ray specialists have become expert in interpreting the films. This, along with the fact that there is an approximate 15 percent error (no greater than the percentage of error of physician-interpretation after examining a breast with a lump in it) in diagnosis even when the films are interpreted by mammograph experts, limits the value of the technique. Though still a valuable tool, this indicates that mammography must be used only in conjunction with careful manual examination by a physician who is an expert in breast diseases. Also, too many women refuse to undergo either biopsy or local excision of a lump when they are informed that their mammogram is normal. This can be a tragic mistake if the patient happens to be one of the 15 out of 100 breast cancer cases in which the mammogram fails to demonstrate the cancer! (It can also err 15 percent in reverse: it can show cancer when none, in fact, exists.)

Mammography therefore is of greatest value when it shows a suspiciously cancerous area. Such a finding positively indicates the need for prompt biopsy. Mammography is of least value when a mammogram is negative, yet a cancer is present—and the reason for arguments recently that the overall effect of mammography has been harmful because women who formerly would have been subjected to immediate biopsy are now delaying or not undergoing biopsy.

Obviously, the safest existing procedure is to operate on every localized lump and to submit it for microscopic examination. The accuracy of the microscope and the expertise of the pathologist when he views a section of the lump under his microscope far surpasses that of both mammography and the clinical impression of the very best breast surgeon.

Suspicious areas usually display on the X-ray film or xerogram deposits of calcium, that appear as tiny, stippled dots. When these areas of micro-calcification are associated with a lump, no problem exists about locating and completely excising the site surgically. However, in some cases the calcific deposits are found in a breast without a dominant lump, and this makes location of the site exceedingly difficult at operation. The area must be carefully marked out by the radiologist so that the surgeon will not miss it when he operates. In addition, the surgeon must remove a sufficiently wide area of breast tissue so as to be sure he has included the site spotted on mammography. To be absolutely certain, some surgeons send the tissue they have removed to the X-ray department for filming. After he has been assured that his biopsy includes the area under suspicion, the material is submitted to a frozen section examination by the pathologist. If, on X-raying the biopsy, the calcific deposits are not seen, the surgeon removes an even wider section of breast tissue.

Calcified deposits on mammography do not necessarily indicate the presence of cancer. Benign tumors such as fibroadenomas may become calcified, as may benign papillomas within the milk ducts, sebaceous cysts beneath the skin, and, quite commonly, calcifications may be seen in the walls of tiny arteries or veins of the breast. Experts in mammography know how to distinguish these findings from those suggestive of cancer. However, the need for mammography is not as great in benign disorders (e.g. cysts, fibroadenomas, etc.) as the surgeon can usually make an accurate diagnosis of these lesions merely by feeling the breast.

Among the ingenious new pieces of apparatus that might one day lead to the routine detection of breast cancer before a lump appears is the "density slicer and color coder." The principle of this apparatus is simple. The mammogram would be placed under a television scanning camera. The scanner would examine each tiny portion of the mammogram and determine its photogenic density, dark or light. (This portion of the apparatus is the *density slicing* part.) Then the electrical signal from the scanner is fed through an analyzer that converts each given slice of photographic density to a color—yellow for one shade of density, red for another, green for another—up to a possible 64 different colors. The result is a color mammogram picture in which contrasts stand out boldly and unmistakably, not like the barely visible variations in shades that appear on the ordinary black-and-white mammogram. Hopefully, this would demonstrate a cancer immediately and pinpoint its exact location.

To date, the density slicer and color coder is only in the experimental stage as a detector of breast cancer, but it is already in use in diagnosing brain tumors, goiters, and other medical conditions. The Breast Cancer Task Force of the National Cancer Institute has funded a study of the apparatus in the hope that several years from now, color patterns of breasts will become so standardized that any change in color or outline would point out a cancer as accurately as one would diagnose it on looking at a biopsy under a microscope.

Questions and Answers

Should one go to an X-ray specialist who is an expert in mammography in order to have this type of examination carried out?

Preferably, yes. However, many radiologists are expert in interpreting mammograms even though they do not specialize in the field.

Is mammography expensive?
No.

What is meant by a false positive mammogram?

It is one in which the X ray indicates the presence of a cancer but, in actuality, none exists. This happens in about 15 of 100 cases.

What is meant by a false negative mammogram?

It is one in which the X ray does not show a cancer but, in actuality, one exists. This happens in about 15 out of 100 cases.

If every woman between the ages of 40 and 65 years in the United States were to undergo mammography, how many cancers of the breast would be found?

According to statistics more than 75,000 cases would be found.

Is there any danger from the exposure to X rays from repeated mammography?

No.

What type of calcium deposit is most likely to be associated with a malignancy?

Tiny, stippled dots, sometimes seen clearly only after viewing the X-ray film with a magnifying glass, are more likely to be associated with a cancer. Larger calcifications are more apt to be seen with benign breast disorders.

How long should one wait between mammograms when she is told that an area in the breast requires watching?

Mammographic changes rarely take place quickly. Therefore, a patient should return for a repeat examination in approximately three to four months after the original examination.

Should all women between 35 and 65 years of age undergo routine yearly mammogram X rays?

Yes. The amount of exposure to X rays is insignificant and the information gleaned from mammography may be extremely valuable, if not lifesaving.

18 THERMOGRAPHY

Thermography is a technique in which the heat generated by a particular organ, or part of an organ, is recorded on a special apparatus known as a thermograph. It records with great sensitivity the degree of infrared radiation from the site at which the thermograph is aimed. Recently, successful attempts at diagnosing cancer during its early stages, by applying the thermograph apparatus to the surface of the breast, have been made. The theory underlying this diagnostic modality is that a cancer will generate greater heat than the surrounding normal breast tissue.

Experts in thermography have now gained great experience in its use upon thousands of women with breast disease. They claim that thermography can often detect a cancer before a lump appears and, in some cases, before changes appear on mammography or xeroradiography. The shortcoming of this method of diagnosing breast disorders is that so few physicians have learned to use the apparatus, and so few doctors' offices, diagnostic clinics, and hospitals are equipped with them.

There is little doubt that thermography, as well as other diagnostic aids, will one day be refined to such an extent that it will enable the diagnosis of malignant breast disease soon after its inception. Let us hope that day will be soon.

Questions and Answers

Is thermography very accurate in diagnosing cancer of the breast before a lump can be felt?

It is much less accurate than mammography and is therefore not used as the sole method of arriving at a diagnosis of breast disease.

Is thermography advocated as a routine form of breast examination?
No. It is usually done only at special clinics set up for diagnostic purposes.

Is thermography painful?
No.

Is thermography usually used in conjunction with mammography?
Yes. A thermogram may show a particular spot in the breast that radiates more heat than other areas. This is known as a hot area. The radiologist, aware of this hot area, will concentrate his mammogram at the site, in the hope of discovering the reason for the thermographic findings.

Do tumors other than cancer get confused with cancer on a thermographic examination?
Yes, occasionally, as benign tumors may also produce a hot reading.

If thermography shows an area suspicious of a tumor but the mammogram is negative, should a patient undergo biopsy?
Every possible lead to the discovery of a breast tumor in its earliest stages of development should be followed. Therefore, if thermography reveals the same hot area on more than one occasion, the woman would be wise to have the site biopsied by a surgeon.

19 TRANS-ILLUMINATION

Transillumination is the passage of a powerful light beam into the substance of the breast. It must be carried out in a darkened room, after the examining physician has accommodated his eyes to the darkness.

Quite a few physicians who treat large numbers of patients with breast disorders become adept at interpreting shadows seen on transillumination, but the method has limited usefulness. It is often possible through transillumination to distinguish between a cyst and a solid tumor, but it is not frequently possible to tell with any degree of certainty whether the solid tumor is benign or malignant. The main use of transillumination, then, is to add to the clinical impression gained from manual examination of the breast. If a physician thinks the borders of a lump are smooth in contour, he may be able to verify this impression with transillumination. Conversely, the light may throw an irregular shadow along the border of a lump, leading the examiner toward the impression that a malignant growth is present.

In distinguishing a cyst from a solid tumor, one notes that the light passes more readily through the fluid of the cyst than it does through the tissues of a solid mass.

Transillumination is not a substitute for mammography as it cannot spot a tumor that is too small to feel manually.

Questions and Answers

Is transillumination usually carried out along with manual examination of the breast?
Yes.

How accurate is transillumination in distinguishing a cyst from a solid tumor?
It is fairly accurate, but the diagnosis will depend more on the manual palpation of the lump.

20 ANESTHESIA IN BREAST SURGERY

Women want assurances that pain will be kept to a minimum before, during, and after their breast operation. Toward this end, they usually discuss the type of anesthesia they will receive, and they are quick to inform the surgeon that they do not want local anesthesia. The surgeon will tell them that local anesthesia is rarely employed in breast surgery unless the procedure is exceptionally minor, or in the rare patient whose general condition is so poor that she cannot be given an inhalation anesthesia.

An important phase of anesthesia is preoperative evaluation and premedication. The anesthesiologist will scan the patient's past history and present medical record to note findings that might influence the choice of anesthetic agent. Having decided on the technique to be used, he will discuss it with his patient and allay any fears that may exist. Occasionally, a woman will inform the anesthesiologist that she had a bad experience at a previous operation with a particular anesthetic agent. The anesthesiologist will take this information into account although it is well known that allergies or sensitivities to a particular anesthetic agent are exceedingly infrequent.

To smooth the entire operative experience, the anesthesiologist will order pills or an injection the night before to ensure a good night's sleep, and narcotics just prior to embarking for the operating room in the morning. Other medications are also prescribed to dry up bronchial secretions before the administration of the inhalation anesthesia. As mentioned previously, the patient can aid her own anesthesia and postoperative course by discontinuing smoking and drinking for several days prior to entering the hospital. Also, patients should be advised to notify their surgeons should any respiratory infection or cough develop. These conditions may require postponement of the operation for a few days, as they often lead to postanesthetic lung complications.

Some women object to removing dentures and nail polish before going to surgery. Both these procedures are necessary, despite the fact that they conflict with a patient's desire to look her best when she greets her surgeon in the operating room. Dentures can be broken during the induction of anesthesia and on rare occasions, when not removed beforehand, have been known to get loose and obstruct the air passages. During anesthesia, the anesthesiologist often looks at the color of the fingernails to see if they are the desired pink tint. This affords him a check on whether sufficient oxygen is being supplied along with the anesthetic agent. Naturally, this information is denied the anesthesiologist when the nails are colored by a polish.

Older people may remember the terrifying experience of years ago when a mask was clamped over their face and, if necessary, they were held down by nurses and doctors while ether was poured onto the mask. Others recall the pain and shock of a long needle being thrust into their back for a spinal anesthesia. Fortunately, these practices have long faded and modern anesthesia can be a rather comforting experience. The premedication puts the patient into a happy, drowsy state, or complete sleep can be attained by a simple injection of one of the barbiturates, such as Pentothal, into a small vein in the hand or arm. By such methods of induction are the initial steps of anesthesia accomplished, without excitement or much ado.

There are several gases used today in conjunction with the sleep-inducing Pentothal or similar agent. These include nitrous oxide, cyclopropane, halothane, or ether. The gases are not inhaled until the patient is asleep from the intravenous medication. All anesthetics for inhalation are used in combination with oxygen, the amount of oxygen being maintained, at all times, at a concentration greater than the air we breathe.

All anesthesia, when given by well-trained anesthesiologists, has a high safety factor, but anesthesia for breast disease is exceptionally safe.

In those patients who will undergo biopsy or the local removal of a cyst or tumor, a light anesthesia can be given. The operation will be of short duration and the patient will be awake within a few minutes after the anesthesia has been discontinued. Those women who will undergo breast removal and those who will have an extensive plastic operation are given endotracheal anesthesia. This means that the anesthetic agent is administered through a tube that is inserted through the mouth into the trachea, or windpipe. The patient is sound asleep during the entire procedure. Endotracheal anesthesia affords better control of the amount of anesthetic agent that is given and permits better control of respirations during a prolonged operative procedure. Once in a while a postoperative patient will complain of a sore throat and may cough a little bloody sputum as a result of irritation caused by the endotracheal tube. These symptoms will subside within a few days without permanent damage to the throat or trachea.

Patients on whom major breast surgery has been done may not awaken from the anesthesia for an hour or more afterward. They are cared for during this period in the Recovery Room, and are not released to their rooms until fully awake.

Questions and Answers

Who administers the anesthesia?

In most hospitals throughout this country, physicians give the anesthesia. When physician-anesthesiologists are not available, specially trained nurses render the anesthesia.

Do women ever talk and give away secrets as they go under or emerge from anesthesia?

They may talk, but they do not "give away secrets." This is a common misconception.

If a woman has had difficulty with a previous anesthesia does this mean she is apt to have a similar reaction to a subsequent anesthesia?

No. There is no such thing as a patient having an inherent tendency to react badly to all anesthesia. The fact that something went amiss at a previous anesthesia does not predispose the patient to a similar, subsequent experience.

How does the anesthesiologist know his patient is fully asleep?

There are many tests to make certain that unconsciousness has been attained and that the patient will feel no pain. No one should ever fear that the surgeon will begin the operation too soon.

Are complications from anesthesia for breast surgery seen frequently?

No. They are rare.

21 BEFORE AND AFTER BREAST SURGERY

When anyone learns that she must undergo surgery, no matter how minor it might be, there is always apprehension. When it is breast surgery, the apprehension is exceptionally intense for fear that a malignancy will be found. Immediately, many questions come to mind during the visit to the surgeon, and many more arise later on when the patient has left his office. To allay some of these apprehensions, many of the most asked questions will be answered in the following pages.

Every patient wants to know how necessary the contemplated surgery is, whether it constitutes an emergency, whether it is an optional procedure, and how long a time can be safely permitted to elapse before undergoing the operation. The patient has the right to know these facts and it is incumbent upon the surgeon to give full, forthright answers. The days when doctors consciously withheld important information from their patients have long since passed. The Patient's Bill of Rights entitles her to know all the facts and all the options surrounding her condition.

Patients often want a second opinion before submitting to breast surgery. If the wish is expressed, it should be granted. The surgeon or the family doctor will suggest the name of a consultant. In this connection, it must be realized that honest differences of opinion exist between equally reputable surgeons. One may advise biopsy of a particular lump in the breast whereas another may advise watchful observation of the suspected area. Naturally, the patient tends to heed the advice of the more conservative consultant in the hope of avoiding surgery. Such a decision on the part of the patient can sometimes be the riskier one—no one succumbs to a breast biopsy but one may succumb to a tumor that grows to large proportions during a prolonged period of "watchfulness."

If two competent surgeons disagree on the need to operate on a particular breast lesion, the patient should seek a third opinion. The third surgeon should be informed of the variance in the opinions of the first two surgeons before he conducts his examination and the patient should be prepared beforehand to abide by the third opinion.

In other sections of this book, aids to the diagnoses of breast disease are fully discussed. Wherever the slightest doubt exists as to the exact nature of the condition, the surgeon will recommend mammography or one of the other tests such as xeroradiography or thermography. However, these tests are only guides to appropriate treatment and do not constitute decisive factors in determining the proper course of therapy.

Already mentioned are measures carried out even before the patient enters the hospital that can aid her postoperative course. If a woman is a heavy smoker, she should make every effort to stop during the interval between the decision to enter the hospital and the admission date. This will lead to a smoother anesthesia and will lessen the chances of a postoperative respiratory infection. If she is a heavy drinker, she should discontinue the practice as this, too, will lessen the incidence of anesthetic and respiratory complications. In addition, women about to undergo surgery should see that they get plenty of rest and sleep for the days preceding hospitalization. An overworked, tired woman is more prone to develop a postoperative infection or other complication. Also, patients who are on medications for unrelated conditions should ask their surgeon whether to continue or discontinue their use before and during hospitalization. As examples, a diabetic must know if dosages of insulin or antidiabetic pills must be altered because of the operation; a woman with high blood pressure must know if she should discontinue her medication during the preoperative days. (Many anesthesiologists advise patients to stop drugs to lower blood pressure until well after the operation.)

Women are almost always concerned about undergoing a breast

operation during their menstrual period, and they should be assured that menstruation in no way interferes with this type of surgery.

Upon entering the hospital for breast surgery, the same routine care is given as for other surgical patients. A chest X ray and electrocardiogram will be performed, urinalysis and blood counts will be done, the blood will be typed and cross-matched for possible transfusion if breast removal is eventually carried out, and chemical analysis of the blood will be undertaken. However, if a mammogram has not been done prior to admission, it may be performed in the hospital on the day preceding surgery.

The night before surgery, the hair on the breast and in the underarm area will be shaved, and the patient will be given a sleeping pill to ensure a good night's rest. If the bowels have not been thoroughly emptied the day before surgery, an enema will be given. If the operation is scheduled for the next morning, all solids and fluids will be withheld after midnight. On the morning of surgery preanesthetic medications are given so that the patient enters the operating room in a drowsy, relaxed state.

The family should never judge the seriousness of the operation by the length of time the patient is in the operating suite. It is customary to send for patients some time in advance of the actual time of the operation. Anesthesiologists often make additional preparations that can occupy one-half to one hour. Occasionally, the surgeon is delayed because he had to take more time with a preceding case than he had expected, thus delaying the time of beginning his next operation. And lastly, in most hospitals, the patient is sent from the operating room to a recovery room until she has fully emerged from the anesthesia. This may take from one to several hours, depending on the amount of anesthetic that has been administered and the patient's individual response to the anesthetic agent.

Breast operations seldom endanger the life of the patient. Operative mortality, even with the most radical type of mastectomy, is so rare that it must be classified as secondary to cardiac arrest, an anesthetic accident, or to the exceptionally poor general condition of the patient. Although extensive breast removal or extensive plastic operations are sometimes accompanied by considerable blood loss, this loss can be readily overcome by transfusions.

A woman who has undergone biopsy or local removal of a cyst or tumor needs little special postoperative care. She is permitted to eat and to get out of bed later in the day of surgery or, at the latest, the day following surgery. By the second postoperative day, the woman can usually be discharged from the hospital.

A woman who has undergone breast removal or a major plastic operation to reduce the size of the breast will require considerable postoperative attention. If she can afford it, special nurses for two to three days will tide her over the most uncomfortable period. Although patients subjected to major breast operations are permitted out of bed the day after surgery, they may require intravenous infusions and dressing changes, which are best attended by specially trained nurses. A hospital stay of one week to ten days is not unusual following mastectomy or a breast reduction procedure. Those who have been operated on for breast augmentation require only a few days in the hospital.

Pain is not an outstanding symptom of breast surgery during the immediate postoperative period. Although the breast is an extremely sensitive organ, its sensitivity to pain is not great and few patients complain much about this. But it does not hold true for the convalescent period after breast removal. Pain in the wound area, the shoulder, and the arm is often persistent and severe, but the time of onset is usually delayed until a month or two after recovery from the surgery.

Wound dressings in minor surgical cases are not particularly painful, even if the incision is near the nipple. Removal of sutures is a simple matter, slightly uncomfortable, but not productive of serious pain. Dressings after breast removal or major plastic surgery may result in considerable discomfort, especially when drains have been inserted or when serum collects beneath the skin. A pain-relieving drug or a narcotic will bring relief within a short time after the dressing has been changed. In minor breast surgical cases, sutures can be removed anywhere from the fifth to eighth postoperative day and in major cases, anywhere from the seventh to the fourteenth day.

As for the serum that collects beneath the skin, it can be readily withdrawn by inserting a needle attached to a syringe, or removed by inserting a clamp into the wound. Neither procedure is painful. Often serum collects a second or third time, until finally the wound heals solidly.

Some surgeons hook up their postoperative mastectomy patients to a water suction apparatus near the bedside in order to facilitate serum drainage. If this is done, the patient may be somewhat limited in her movements for the first few days after surgery. Other surgeons insert a specially devised suction apparatus known as a Hemovac, which patients can wear around the waist during the first few postoperative days.

Patients should be cautioned about an empty space left in the breast after the removal of a lump. To fill in this gap, the surgeon sews together the breast tissues that surround the lump. *When healing takes place, the patient may feel a thickening that, indeed, can be larger than the original lump for which she was operated!* This does not mean that the surgeon failed to remove the lump. The thickening is caused by the normal healing process, which lays down fibrous tissue along the line where the breast has been repaired. This lump will disappear gradually over a period of several months.

A number of uncomfortable symptoms—common to most postoperative patients—which affect the woman whose breast has undergone surgery are:

1. Nausea and vomiting, usually secondary to anesthesia, to the administration of a narcotic, or to eating or drinking too much too soon after surgery.

2. Headache, usually secondary to anesthesia or to a medication given during surgery.

3. Dizziness and weakness, experienced by an extraordinary number of women who have had breast surgery. These symptoms may be severe even after the most minor type of operation, suggesting that the reactions are more psychological than physical. It is not at all uncommon for these patients to complain of dizziness and weakness for several weeks after breast surgery and it is the duty of the surgeon to reassure them and to lend a sympathetic ear. Tranquilizers are only a moderately effective remedy; certainly, they do not take the place of considerate medical attention.

Questions and Answers

How soon should an operation be done after it is decided on?

Tumors suspected of harboring malignancy should be done no later than three weeks after the diagnosis has been made. Other lesions should be done within a few weeks after diagnosis.

The sooner any indicated breast operation is performed, the sooner will the patient's anxiety be relieved.

Can breast operations be performed in the office?

In most instances, no. Cysts can be emptied with a needle and syringe in an office but other procedures should be done under general anesthesia in a hospital.

How sure can one be, before surgery, that a lump is not malignant?

In the great majority of cases, a distinction between a malignant and nonmalignant condition can be made before surgery by manual examination of the breast, and by mammography. However, reliance should not be placed on these methods alone. Biopsy, plus microscopic examination of the tissue, is essential to a positive diagnosis.

Will the surgeon be able to tell whether the growth is cancerous while the patient is undergoing surgery?

Yes, because he will submit the tissue he removes to immediate, frozen-section, microscopic examination, carried out by the surgical pathologist.

What kinds of operations are performed for breast disease?

1. Local excision of a cyst or benign tumor.

2. Radical mastectomy, including removal of the breast, muscles of the chest wall, and lymph glands in the armpit for most cancers.

3. Modified radical mastectomy, in which the breast and lymph nodes in the armpit are removed but the muscles of the chest wall are not removed.

4. Simple mastectomy in which the breast is removed but the muscles of the chest wall and the lymph glands in the armpit are not removed.

5. Excision of the ductal system of the breast in women with potentially malignant tumors of the milk ducts.

6. Subcutaneous mastectomy, involving removal of all of the glandular tissue of the breast while leaving behind the nipple, skin, and subcutaneous tissues. This is reserved for those with recurring cystic disease or intraductal papillomas that are potentially malignant.

7. Excision of the tail of the breast when it is markedly overgrown and causes unusual pain.

How long do breast operations take to perform?

Local excisions take from ten to thirty minutes to perform; breast removal, especially radical procedures, may require from 1½ to 6 hours to complete.

Are breast operations dangerous?

No, but they are serious. Recovery from the operative procedure takes place in almost all cases. Deaths from breast operations are due to the poor general health of the patient or to an anesthetic accident, or cardiac arrest.

Will one require blood transfusions during an operation for removal of the breast?

Some patients do; others don't. It will depend on the amount of blood lost during surgery and the hemoglobin of the patient prior to surgery. One who was anemic prior to surgery is more likely to require a transfusion.

How long does it take a breast wound to heal?

1. Wounds of local excision will heal in 6 to 8 days.
2. Wounds following breast removal or certain types of major plastic surgery may take 8 to 14 days to heal.

Do breast operations disfigure?

Breast removal will, but scars of local excision usually cause no disfigurement. See "Scars from Breast Surgery."

Will the scar be visible when a bathing suit or evening dress is worn?

No. Most breast scars, even those for radical removal, are so positioned that they are hidden from view when the woman wears a bathing suit or evening dress.

How long does it take to convalesce from breast operations?

After local excision, a patient can go back to work within a few days. After breast removal or a major plastic procedure, a month may be required for convalescence. However, some women require several weeks to convalesce from a breast operation no matter how minor the procedure.

Must an operation on the breast affect one's sex life?

It should not in any physical way.

22 SCARS FROM BREAST SURGERY

A considerable number of patients hesitate to accept breast surgery for fear that the resulting scar will cause disfigurement. These women would rather risk the danger of retaining a lump in their breast in order to avoid an unsightly scar. And yet in the great majority of cases, breast scars are minimal or invisible after the passage of a few months' time.

A sufficient number of breast lesions occur near enough to the outer circumference of the nipple to enable an incision to be made in a semicircular fashion between the nipple and its surrounding skin. This incision is known as a periareolar incision. For some unknown reason, the tissues of the nipple heal with an almost invisible scar. After the incision is made, the surgeon lifts up the skin and dissects under it and outward toward the cyst or tumor. After the lump has been removed and bleeding has been controlled, the skin incision is closed.

Some lesions are so far away from the nipple that an incision must be made directly over them. In these cases, too, the surgeon tries to place the incision so that a minimal scar will result. He may be able to reach a lump in the upper outer part of the breast by making the incision near the armpit. This maneuver may result in the scar being hidden by the arm or the folds of the skin near the armpit. Lesions in the lower part of the breast can sometimes be reached through an incision in the underfold of the breast. The incision is called inframammary. The resultant scar in this type of case may be totally hidden by the breast itself.

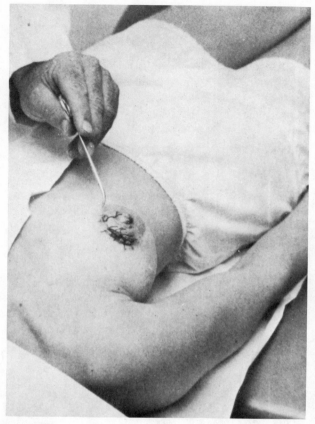

Most benign breast tumors can be removed through an incision surrounding the nipple. This will result in little or no scarring.

Radial incisions made directly over the site of disease tend to leave the most visible scars, but even these tend to blanch within a year or two, leaving no visible disfigurement.

Patients frequently ask whether removal of a lump will result in an indentation and a loss of the rounded contour of the breast. They can be assured that this will not happen as the normal breast tissue surrounding the site of excision fills in the gap left by the removal of the lump. Normal contours are restored in almost all cases unless an extraordinary amount of tissue has been removed.

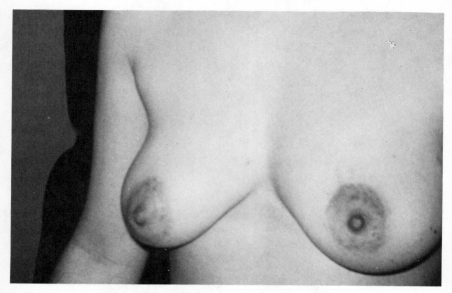

Both of these patients had benign tumors removed through periareolar incisions made in the area surrounding the upper portion of the nipples. Two years later the scars are practically invisible.

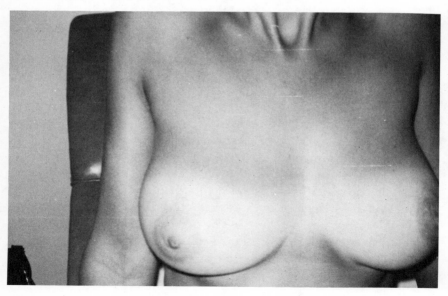

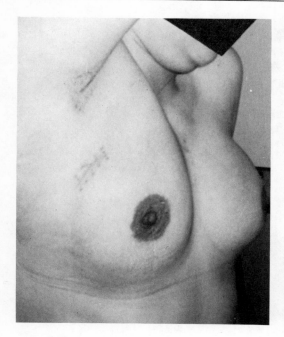

The scar for the removal of the tail of the breast is made far out toward the armpit and cannot be seen when the arm is lowered. It will fade as time passes.

It must be understood that the surgeon is always more interested in removing the entire diseased area than in obtaining a good cosmetic result. For this reason, he will not sacrifice thoroughness for fear of creating an unsightly scar.

Scars from mastectomy, whether from a simple breast removal or from a radical mastectomy, are not pretty. They extend from the edge of the rib cage in an upward and outward direction toward the shoulder and armpit. But, here, too, the surgeon is always conscious of the need to place his incision so that the patient will, after recovery, be able to wear a bathing suit or evening dress without showing the scar. This can be accomplished in almost every case. As a result, no one can see that a woman has undergone mastectomy unless she is undressed.

Incisions in plastic operations, when placed around the nipple or beneath the breast, leave minimal scars. In operations to reduce the size of the breast, scars may eventually result. However, the aim in this type of case is to produce more attractive contours, and the penalty of so doing is to create visible breast scars.

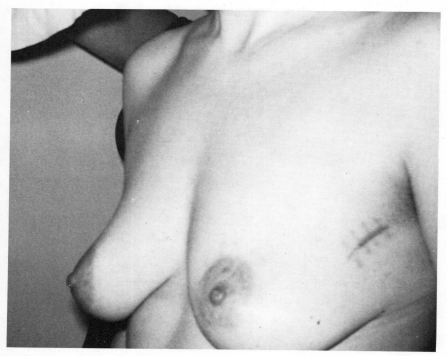

Radial scars such as this one far out on the breast not infrequently leave noticeable, overgrown scars. However, even this will fade somewhat in time.

Questions and Answers

Are scars from the ordinary breast biopsy disfiguring?

No. They are usually linear scars between one and two inches long that blanch out over a period of several months and become almost invisible. Few biopsy wounds lead to disfigurement.

Why is it that some scars due to surgery heal with a very fine line whereas others are overgrown and unsightly?

People have various reactions to surgical incisions. Some people heal with just a thin white line as the end result, others heal with thick, overgrown, broad scars. The surgeon has no influence on the type of scar a patient will ultimately develop.

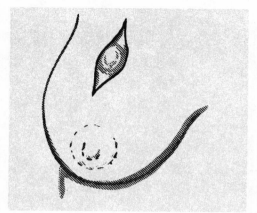

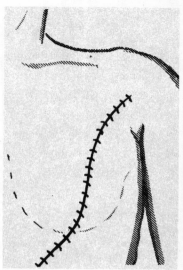

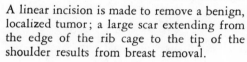

A linear incision is made to remove a benign, localized tumor; a large scar extending from the edge of the rib cage to the tip of the shoulder results from breast removal.

Can scars ever be removed if they are ugly?

Yes, if they are overgrown or large. If, however, the scar is a keloid, that is, abnormally overgrown, it may be replaced by another keloid that can exceed the original scar in size.

What is a radial incision?

One that is made perpendicularly to the nipple. It has the direction of a spoke in a wheel.

Does X-ray or cobalt treatment scar the breast?

No, but it may cause small blood vessels to become more prominent in the skin.

Are there any medications that can be applied to a scar to make it shrink and become less prominent?

No.

How long may it take a scar on the breast to reach its smallest size?

A year or two may elapse before a breast scar reaches its ultimate appearance.

23 PLASTIC SURGERY ON THE BREAST

In several other chapters attractiveness of the breasts has been mentioned. Most women make special efforts to present their best possible contours. Often women who think their breasts are unattractive and look for ways to improve them are hoodwinked into buying fraudulent devices such as "bust developers" and "exercisers" to strengthen "the muscles" of their breasts so that they become more upright and firmer to the touch. Other women seek hormone ointments, tablets, or injections to enlarge their breasts and to help them retain their youthful appearance and fullness. Curiously, some women with small breasts are sometimes persuaded to have expensive massage treatments to augment their size whereas others take similar massage treatments to reduce their oversized breasts. "Spot reducing" therapy is frequently undertaken by gullible women whose desire to lose weight in the breast area the easy way is so great that they abandon common sense.

We've already discussed the futility of these measures for the purpose of beautifying the breasts and that the best course to follow, short of plastic surgery, is to maintain a normal body weight, exercise regularly to promote good muscle tone, and to wear a good supporting brassiere. Also, repeated overexposure to the sun should be avoided as this will cause the skin of the exposed portion of the breast to age prematurely.

The desire for breast beautification is not limited to any particular age group. Young and old alike display great interest in the possibilities

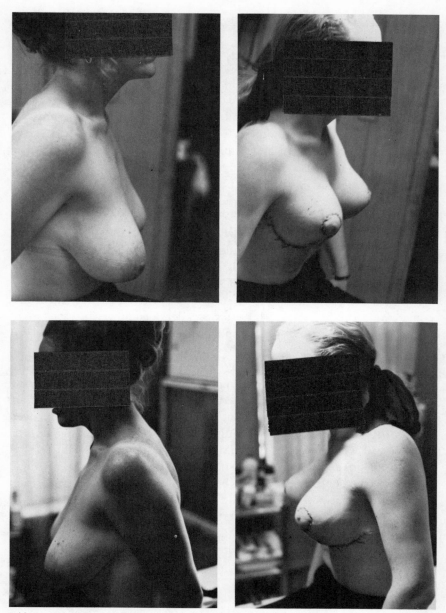

Before and after: Breasts reduced through plastic surgery.

of help through plastic surgery, and it should not be denied them on the basis of age. The most important consideration is the type and extent of the breast deformity, for one should never undergo major surgery for a minor defect. An equally important consideration is the emotional stability of the patient for it has been found that insecure, maladjusted, unstable women are usually poor candidates for breastplasty. They tend to expect that the operation will somehow cure emotional ills that are unrelated to the fact that their breasts are too small or too large.

Plastic surgeons, if their practices are extensive, soon become quite familiar with the psychological problems of their patients. Many have become so expert in diagnosing the breast-related emotional problems of their intended patients that they will know beforehand who should or should not be subjected to breast reduction or breast augmentation. When in doubt, most plastic surgeons will refer their patients for a psychiatric evaluation prior to proceeding with surgery.

Plastic surgery on the breasts has developed into a fine art within recent years. The breasts can be made smaller, pendulous breasts can be elevated, ugly scars can be excised, and small breasts can be made to appear larger. Most of these operations must be considered major procedures, not in the risk to life that is involved, but in the skill necessary to achieve satisfactory results. Breastplasty should not be performed indiscriminately on capricious women who wish to correct minor sagging, to reduce slight enlargement, or to enlarge breasts that are near normal in size. Moreover, this type of surgery should be performed only by a skilled plastic surgeon who has had wide experience in the field.

The main indications for plastic operations on the breast are:

1. Marked enlargement. Such breasts are heavy, unsightly, and exert a constant, painful pull on the shoulders, with severe indentations into the skin of the shoulders by the brassiere straps.

I know of few abnormalities that concern women, especially adolescent females, more than oversized breasts. We are referring to females of normal or near-normal weight with exceptionally large breasts. Markedly obese females with extremely large breasts are not candidates for plastic surgery.

2. Hypertrophy of one or both breasts. There are two types of hypertrophy, or overgrown breasts, namely, that occurring during adolescence, and that associated with pregnancy.

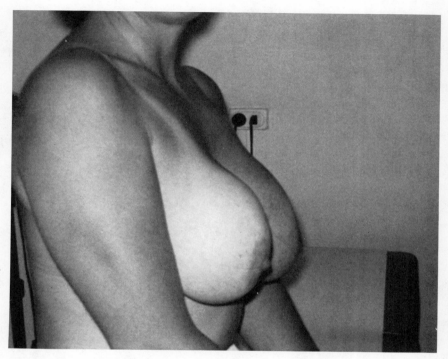

Breast enlargement, three years following the augmentation operation. The patient had relatively small, sagging breasts prior to the insertion of silastic bags containing an inert fluid.

Although breast hypertrophy is thought to involve a hormone imbalance, this theory is not completely accepted since the condition may involve one breast only. If the overgrowth were glandular in origin, one would expect that both breasts would be afflicted.

Hypertrophy associated with pregnancy is considered of hormonal origin. It is well to reserve breast reduction in these patients until childbearing is completed. A well-executed plastic operation may be wasted if the patient has additional pregnancies again associated with pathological breast hypertrophy.

The patient with hypertrophy who seeks surgical care usually has a breast or breasts anywhere from twice to four or five times normal size.

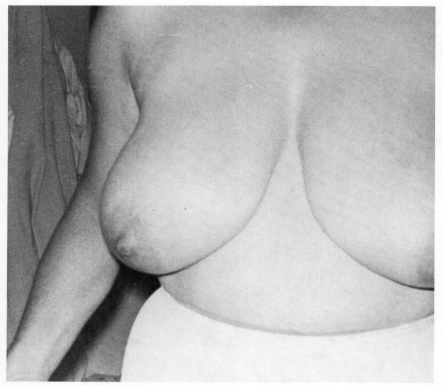

Large pendulous breasts lend themselves well to breastplasty.

Those with slight overgrowths are not candidates for breast plastic operations.

3. Dissimilar breasts. Although there may be some minor disparity in the size of a woman's breasts, major differences in size cause considerable concern and embarrassment. If the disparity is great, equalization of breast size can be effected either by breast reduction of one breast or augmentation of the other.

4. Pendulous breasts. Some breasts may sag 6 to 8 inches below their normal position, even though they are not markedly enlarged. Women who have this condition frequently want it corrected not only because it

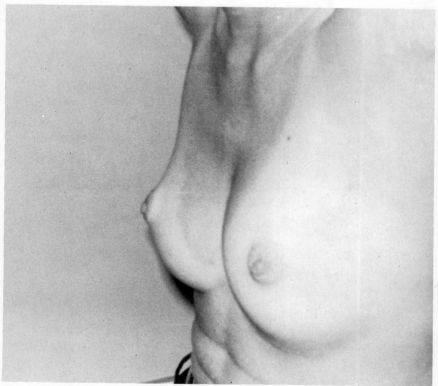

This young lady sought breast augmentation because she thought her breasts were too small. The plastic surgeon rejected her request for surgery.

is unattractive but because the skin underneath such breasts is difficult to keep dry and often becomes irritated.

    5. Underdeveloped or exceptionally small breasts. On occasion, one or both breasts fail to mature, either because of some underlying hormone deficiency or because one has inherited the characteristic of small breasts. An adolescent with one normally developed breast and one undeveloped breast is an unhappy girl who, sooner or later, will seek relief through plastic surgery.

    Most women with small breasts have normal reproductive systems and are just as well developed sexually as their large-breasted counterparts.

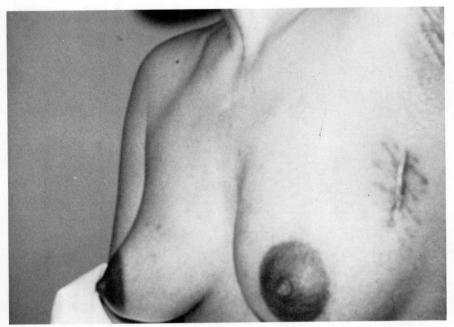

Keloids, or abnormally overgrown scars, sometimes occur. They should be treated conservatively as occasionally their removal leads to an even bigger scar.

They have merely inherited a familial trait of small-breastedness. This knowledge, however, fails to satisfy many young people and as a consequence, they present themselves to the surgeon for an augmentation procedure.

6. Ugly scars, secondary to burns, lacerations, or surgical wounds, can generally be excised and the skin resutured in a manner to give a minimal scar. Breast surgeons can help decrease the incidence of unsightly scars by making their incisions around the nipple (periareolar incisions) whenever possible. However, if the tumor or cyst is far out from the nipple, this type of incision may not be feasible.

Keloids tend to be more prevalent in the upper outer portion of the breast. Their cause is not known and a woman who wants a keloid removed must be warned that there is a very high incidence—from 30 to 50 percent—of recurrence, and that the new keloid may be even larger than the original one. Superficial X-ray treatment to the wound area carried out during the immediate postoperative period cuts down somewhat on the incidence of recurrent keloids.

7. Recently, plastic surgeons, by inserting cone-shaped silicone bags filled with fluid, have reconstructed the appearance of a breast on the chest wall of patients who have undergone mastectomy. This procedure has not been utilized very greatly to date, for fear that the extensive skin mobilization on the chest wall may activate dormant, residual cancer cells in the area. Others reject the operation on the grounds that the plastic implant might hide a local recurrence of tumor should it develop.

However, if the breast surgeon who has performed the mastectomy concurs, the plastic procedure certainly can help to restore more normal contours.

8. Psychological disturbance. As mentioned previously, the breast plastic surgeon hesitates before operating on an emotionally insecure patient. On the other hand, from time to time, a surgeon will receive a referral from a psychiatrist who believes breastplasty will benefit his patient. These are rare instances. More commonly, the surgeon encounters a patient with a relatively minor breast deformity with a major psychological disturbance. In this connection, a good number of young women attribute their inability to find a mate to their oversized or pendulous breasts. Because of self-consciousness, they abstain from participation in many activities and refuse to wear bathing suits or revealing evening gowns. These people require psychotherapy rather than plastic surgery.

There are several different techniques for the surgical correction of enlarged and pendulous breasts. Each has its advocates, and each is a good operation when performed carefully and expertly. Plastic operations on the breast must be performed in the hospital under general anesthesia. Whenever possible, both breasts are operated on at the same time. The procedure often takes 1½ to 2½ hours for each breast. It is important, therefore, that the patient be in good general health before undergoing this type of surgery.

The essential principle underlying these operations is to preserve the blood supply to the nipple and the blood supply of the skin flaps. In performing these procedures, the nipple is encircled with an incision but is left attached to the underlying breast tissue. Skin flaps are elevated from

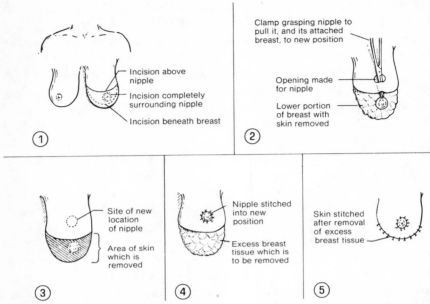

The surgical procedure for making a breast smaller and reshaping it so that the nipple is in normal position.

the underlying breast tissue by undermining the skin in an outward direction from the nipple. The excess breast tissue is then cut off. The remaining section of breast, with nipple attached, is elevated to a higher location on the chest wall and the nipple is brought through a snug-fitting hole that is fashioned in the upper skin flap. Next, the excess skin from the lower part of the breast is cut away and all skin edges are sutured together neatly.

Drains are inserted into the wound to permit the exit of serum, which usually forms within a day or two. The drains are removed several days later but the stitches are permitted to remain in place for 10 to 12 days postoperatively. The patient may get out of bed on the first or second postoperative day and may leave the hospital, with stitches still in place, anywhere from the fifth to the eighth day after surgery.

The most frequently encountered complication of breastplasty in former years was postoperative infection. Such infection sometimes destroyed the cosmetic result and left the patient with areas that would drain pus for months afterward. Fortunately, improvement in surgical techniques and the proper use of antibiotic drugs have minimized this danger. Today, excellent results are being obtained in the overwhelming majority of cases.

For breast augmentation there are the plastic sacs (silastic) containing an inert fluid. These are made in a convex, round shape to conform to the desired size of the breast. There are two methods most popularly used to carry out breast augmentation. In one method, a transverse incision about 3 inches is made below the breast and a pouch is fashioned by the surgeon underneath the breast tissue on the chest wall. After all bleeding has been meticulously controlled, the empty plastic sac is slipped into this pouch and is inflated with an appropriate amount of salt solution, thus elevating the overlying breast tissue and giving the appearance of enlargement. The skin incision beneath the breast is then closed.

The second method of breast augmentation is done in the same way except that the incision is made around the nipple. After fashioning a pouch under the breast tissue, the surgeon inserts the plastic bag, fills it with fluid, and closes the skin. This procedure has a better cosmetic result as the incision above the nipple is barely visible after it heals. However, it is not possible, with this method, to ensure absolute control of bleeding. As a consequence, the chances for rejection of the plastic bag are somewhat greater because of a blood collection about the sac or because of secondary infection.

Breast augmentation procedures should be performed only by expert plastic surgeons under the most rigid aseptic conditions. Although the operations are simple to carry out, not all patients can accept the large sac; their tissues may fail to encapsulate it. In such cases, a draining sinus will develop and the sac will have to be removed. A second attempt can be made several months later if all inflammation has subsided, but the chances are greater that a similar rejection of the inserted sac will take place.

Questions and Answers

Are exercises effective in elevating sagging breasts?

No. However, to retain a good figure, physical exercise should be performed regularly.

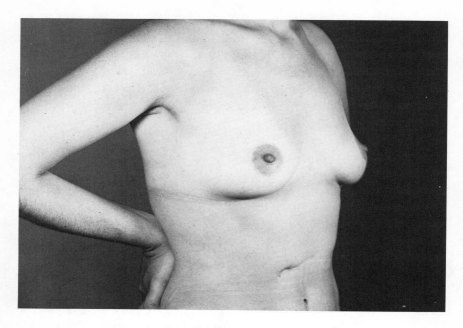

Before and after pictures of breasts made to appear larger by inserting a plastic implant through a periareolar incision.

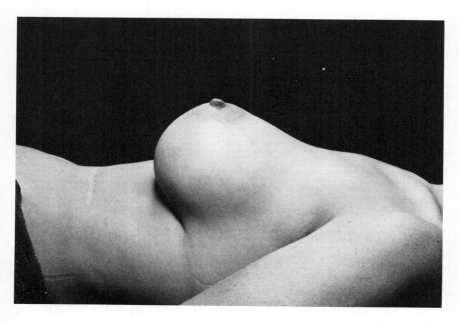

Will rubbing the breasts with ointments containing estrogen or the taking of estrogen tablets or injections enlarge and make the breast feel firmer?

Yes, in some women, but the effect lasts only so long as one uses the hormone. Moreover, harm can result from using estrogens without a physician's advice.

Is it safe to inject silicone under the skin to fill out the breast?

No. Silicone injections may be conducive to tumor formation within the breast.

Is the injection of silicone beneath the skin of the breast legal?

No. In most states, it is considered malpractice.

Can silicone, once injected, be removed from the tissues?

This is exceedingly difficult to do as the silicone spreads throughout all the tissues and does not become encapsulated.

Is it ever necessary to remove a breast that has become involved in tumor formation as a result of silicone injections?

Yes. This must be done to save the patient's life if the silicone-induced tumor is of a malignant nature.

Can constant use of an uplift brassiere elevate the breasts?

Unfortunately, only when the brassiere is worn.

How important is body weight in retaining good breast contour?

It is very important. Both overweight and underweight breasts tend to sag.

Are most enlarged breasts due to overgrowth of gland tissue or to overweight?

In the majority of cases, oversized breasts are due to obesity, not to excessive glandular tissue within the breast.

Do hypertrophied breasts occur mostly in stout women?

No. Since the hypertrophy is due to increased amounts of glandular tissue, it has nothing to do with the weight of the individual.

When is it best to undergo breastplasty?

Young unmarried women with a marked deformity and a marked psychological disturbance occasioned by the breasts may be operated upon, if clearance for surgery has been given by psychiatric evaluation. However, more satisfactory results will follow if surgery is done after women are finished having children.

Do plastic operations interfere with sensations in the breast?
No.

Is pregnancy permissible after a breastplasty?
Yes.

Do the breasts swell during menstrual periods after these operations?
The breasts will react postoperatively the same as they did before the operation.

Can a woman nurse a child after these operations?
Yes, in those cases in which the nipple has been left attached to its underlying breast tissue.

Are breast plastic operations exceptionally painful?
No.

Are there cases where only one breast is enlarged?
Yes, but this is not very common.

Is it more difficult to diagnose the presence of a tumor or cyst after breast reduction has been performed?
Slightly more difficult.

Will making a breast smaller in any way influence the subsequent development of a cyst or tumor?
No.

Should a woman have plastic surgery on her breasts even though a psychiatrist advises against it?
This is extremely unwise.

Does the presence of a plastic sac alter the overlying breast tissue?

There may be some compression of it, but no real alteration takes place.

Will there be alteration in the feel of the breast after the insertion of a plastic sac?

Yes, despite the fact that the sacs being used today are a great improvement over those of several years ago. There is not a completely natural feel to the breast after this type of surgery. The breast may feel too firm, or the edge of the sac, particularly in a thin woman, might be felt.

Is a breast with an implant more sensitive to pain or more tender than normal?

No.

Must augmented breasts with implants be treated gently during love play?

No. They should be treated normally. A well-adjusted, encapsulated implant cannot be damaged by breast participation in lovemaking.

If a woman is dissatisfied with the appearance of her breast following the insertion of a plastic implant, can she have it removed?

Yes, but she must understand that the breast will sag inordinately and have a flat, flabby appearance.

Will the breast always feel flat and flabby following the removal of a breast implant?

Yes, for a certain period of time. In younger women the stretched skin of the breast retains a greater amount of elastic tissue and the chances for it to contract and return to a more normal appearance are greater. In older women whose skin has lost elasticity, the breast may sag and appear flabby permanently.

Are chemicals usually given to combat the rejection of a breast implant?

Chemicals used to overcome rejection of breast implants have not been used as their toxic effects are too dangerous. Such medications may have a damaging effect on the white blood cells of the body.

Will a breast implant have to be removed if a patient subsequently develops a cyst or benign tumor of the overlying breast?

No. Since the breast tissue lies superficial to the implant, it is possible to remove the cyst or tumor without touching the implant.

How advisable is it to have a plastic implant following breast removal?

In all probability it is best to make certain that the tumor will not return before undergoing this procedure. Most surgeons believe that a period of five to ten years should elapse between the time of breast removal for a malignant tumor and the conclusion that there will be no recurrence. For this reason it would seem best not to disturb the area until this period of time has elapsed.

Will the breast look normal if it is constructed from a flat chest wall?

No, but it will give the appearance of a protuberance, and if the woman is clothed, it may look quite well.

Is breast reconstruction more feasible when the opposite breast is of small size?

Yes, it is much more difficult to reconstruct a large breast than a small one.

Are operations done to cure inverted nipples?

Not usually, but the nipple can be undermined surgically, thus cutting tissue fibers that have exerted an inward pull on the nipple.

How successful is removal of an ugly scar from a previous breast operation?

Fairly successful, but in some cases the new scar will be just as ugly as the original one. However, plastic surgeons are more likely to get the best cosmetic result when excising an old scar.

How soon can one operate on keloids in a breast scar?

A period of approximately two years should elapse between the formation of the original keloid and reoperation to excise it.

Are breasts ever removed solely because they are hypertrophied?
Yes. In older women with markedly enlarged breasts, simple removal may be advisable instead of a complicated plastic operation.

Are blood transfusions necessary after plastic surgery on the breast?
No.

Should special brassieres be worn after breast plastic operations?
Not permanently, but a snug-fitting brassiere should be worn for several weeks after surgery.

How long do wounds following breastplasty take to heal?
Seven to twelve days.

Are the results of breastplasty usually permanent?
Yes, although normal aging tends to cause all breasts to lose their youthful contours. Also, if the patient gains or loses an inordinate amount of weight, she may dissipate much of the good results.

Do the breasts tend to regrow after having been reduced in size?
Not usually, unless the patient becomes very stout.

Do the breasts tend to sag again after being elevated?
Not for many years, unless there is marked weight gain.

How soon after surgery can one do the following?

Bathe	10 to 14 days
Housework	3 to 4 weeks
Resume physical exercise	4 to 5 weeks
Resume sexual relations	4 weeks

Is it permissible to do plastic surgery on the breast during the menstrual period?
Yes, this can be done but since the breast is usually engorged during the menstrual period, the surgeon may encounter certain increased bleeding. For this reason, it is preferable to operate shortly after menstruation has stopped.

Can women in their fifties or sixties undergo plastic surgery on the breasts?

Yes, if they so desire and if a surgical indication is present. The age of the woman is not a very important factor.

Do the wounds heal just as well in women who are in their fifties and sixties?

Yes.

Should a woman who has had surgery to enlarge her breasts go for periodic breast examinations?

Yes, this is particularly important as there is an alteration in the feel of the breast that overlies the plastic sac that has been inserted. It is necessary to go to an expert in breast surgery to make sure that no tumor exists within the substance of the breast.

24 THE NIPPLES AND NIPPLE DISCHARGE

The nipples are frequently the site of abnormalities, disorders, and disease. Among the most important of these are:

Congenital deformities. The most common birth anomaly, inherited through the genes, is the supernumerary or accessory nipple, seen in approximately 1 to 2 percent of all births. These structures, found in pairs or singly, are usually seen on the chest wall beneath the true breast or in the upper abdominal region. Most accessory nipples are in a line with the normal nipples but in a minority of cases they are located on the breast itself or in or near the armpit. Extra nipples occur just as often in males as they do in females. As puberty progresses, the accessory nipple may enlarge somewhat. Sometimes, there is breast tissue beneath the accessory nipple but more often true breast tissue is lacking.

Along with other birth deformities of the chest is the absence of one or both breasts. This is an extremely rare deformity, but when it does occur, it affects females more often than males. More commonly, one breast rather than both are missing. Absence of a breast is known as amastia. Until recently, women with an absent nipple (usually associated with an absent breast) received little or no help for their deformity. Today, plastic surgeons are sometimes able to insert a silicone sac beneath the skin of the chest and to utilize a piece of the nipple from the opposite

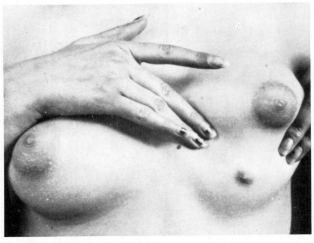

Supernumerary nipple with underlying breast tissue beneath the left breast.

breast as a graft to replace the missing nipple. Results will depend largely on the patient's ability to accept the plastic implant.

Accessory nipples in a child can be removed easily if their presence disturbs the parents, or if a mature individual with this anomaly finds them unsightly. Simple surgical excision results in a small, transverse, linear scar measuring about 1 inch in length. It can be accomplished readily in infancy, childhood, or in adulthood. The presence of accessory nipples is thought to substantiate the theory that humans have descended from lower forms of animal life.

Inverted nipples. Some women have nipples that turn inward instead of outward. Although this may seem to be a minor defect, it is indeed a major one. Inverted nipples interfere with the ability to nurse an infant and also rob a woman of much of the pleasure she might enjoy from the sexual stimulation of the breast. There are no harmful physical effects of inverted nipples except that they tend to collect debris from secretions emanating from the ducts and are therefore difficult to keep clean. The secretions dry out and cake in the crevices caused by the nipple retraction. Massage is usually ineffective in reversing the position of the nipple even though it is frequently advocated by physicians and obstetricians.

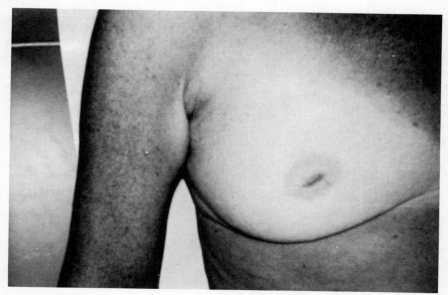

Inverted nipple.

Surgical repair of an inverted nipple is only partly satisfactory as the operation may not result in the nipple's ability to erect. Moreover, repair may require the major milk ducts to be cut across, thus interfering with the ability to nurse. The operation involves a crescentic incision around 50 percent of the outer circumference of the nipple. The nipple is then reflected and lifted up from its underlying connections. Fibrous tissue strands that bind it down are severed, but this does not usually overcome the entire retraction. The retraction, or inversion, is usually caused by a foreshortening of the milk ducts and unless they are cut across, the deformity will not be fully corrected. After thorough mobilization of tissues beneath the entire nipple, it is replaced to its normal position and sutured to the surrounding skin of the breast. Unfortunately, the surgical procedure may sever many of the special nerve fibers contained within this structure.

Cracked nipples, discussed in the pregnancy chapter, are the not uncommon breast complication of pregnancy. The cracked nipple is much the same lesion as a "split lip," and is closely allied to the chapping phenomenon seen so often on the knuckles of the fingers in wintry weather.

Dermatitis. Inflammation of the skin of the nipple is common. The nipple is an active part of the body in that it is vigorously rubbed and suckled during nursing and lovemaking, and is always in moving contact with an overlying brassiere or some item of wearing apparel. Any part of the skin that is subject to repeated friction is likely to become inflamed, and the nipple is no exception. A poorly fitting brassiere can create marked friction and irritation of the nipple within a short period of time. Contact, or allergic, dermatitis is perhaps one of the most provocative causes of nipple inflammation. Many women are sensitive to nylon, Dacron, and other synthetic materials that go to make their brassieres; others may develop dermatitis from a perfume they daub on their nipples or from a powder they employ after bathing.

It is important that nipple dermatitis be distinguished from *Paget's disease,* an ulceration of the nipple secondary to an underlying cancer of the ducts of the breast. Ordinary dermatitis has its onset within a few days' time and responds to adjustment of a poorly fitting brassiere or ointments and the removal of the irritating contact substance (a powder or perfume) within a two-week period. Paget's disease of the nipple requires several months for an ulceration to appear and does not clear up with local treatment. *An absolute distinction between the two lesions can be made by biopsying the nipple and looking under the microscope for cancer cells, which are typical of Paget's disease.*

Whenever a nipple inflammation fails to subside after treatment for two weeks with ointments containing antibiotics or cortisonelike ingredients, or both, a biopsy is indicated. Fortunately, the outlook for patients with Paget's disease is exceptionally good if a biopsy is taken early and definitive surgery is carried out promptly.

Polyps. The nipple is a frequent site for skin polyps. These are small, benign tumors, usually made up of a thin stalk and a rounded head, giving them the appearance of a tiny tennis racquet. They vary in size from 1/4 to 3/4 inches. These tumors have no significance except that they are unsightly and may become irritated by constant rubbing against a brassiere. They can be removed with an electric needle or can merely be tied off with a silk tie. A drop or two of a local anesthetic agent beneath the skin makes this a painless office procedure. Polyps do not tend to recur.

Papilloma. Papilloma of the nipple is a rare benign tumor, arising from the ducts of the breast near their exit on the nipple's surface. As the papilloma grows, it extrudes on to the skin above the nipple. In order to excise this type of tumor at its root, a general anesthesia is required. The papilloma, along with a generous portion of normal surrounding nipple, is excised, and a suture or two is inserted to control bleeding. Remember that nipple tissue heals practically without scar and, therefore, excision of a papilloma will not disfigure the nipple. Papillomas do not become malignant.

Retraction of the nipple, if it comes on during adult life, often signifies the presence of an underlying tumor. The tumor, as it grows, pulls on and may partly invert the nipple. Since retraction is frequently an indication of breast cancer, a woman who notes it should seek immediate medical advice.

Duct ectasia, described elsewhere, is a benign condition that also may give rise to retraction of the nipple.

Infections of the nipple are also described elsewhere. It may follow severe trauma, may result from nursing, or from intense suckling and biting during the foreplay of intercourse. An infection of the nipple tends to spread rapidly along the lymphatic channels into the deeper structure of the breast where it may form an abscess.

Mammary duct fistula has already been described. It is an uncommon condition in which there is a false tract (fistula) or tunnel extending from one of the main milk ducts on to the surface of the nipple near its junction with the surrounding skin. The cause of duct fistula is thought to be an infection that burrows through the wall of the milk duct out into breast tissue and then upward and outward to the surface. The presence of a duct fistula can be noted by the intermittent discharge of a small amount of yellowish or yellowish pink fluid through an opening in the skin off to one side of the nipple. Noticeable nipple disfigurement is rare following removal of a duct fistula.

Nipple Discharge

The ducts of the nipple are normally kept open by the continuous secretion of a small amount of mucus. The secretion is usually invisible as it emerges from the nipple because the amount is so small and much of it evaporates quickly. Also, when women bathe and cleanse their breast area, the material is wiped away in the form of tiny crusts. Some women secrete more than others and, from time to time, they discover a slight discharge on the inside of their brassiere or on their nightgown. Then, too, discharge from the nipple is on the increase because so many women are taking contraceptive pills, or estrogens during or after menopause. The secretions described above are normal and do not indicate the presence of underlying breast disease.

As women are becoming more alert to the danger of breast cancer, and since more women are practicing monthly self-examination, they are showing increased interest and concern about the presence of discharge from their nipples. It might be well here to list the various types of discharge and to comment on their significance:

Colostrum, discussed earlier, the yellow greenish thick material that is the forerunner of milk. It is secreted from the nipple during the last weeks of pregnancy, and when the infant suckles during the first 24 to 48 hours after birth. Colostrum is then replaced by milk.

Milk is not necessary to discuss as a normal secretion of the nursing breast, but in some women, it continues to be secreted for an indefinite period of time after nursing has stopped. The milky secretions in these women are seldom associated with a palpable breast lesion except for the occasional woman who has a galactocele, or milk cyst. However, it is important that they be investigated to exclude the presence of an ovarian or adrenal gland tumor. If none is found, and if the milk secretion is copious and annoying, one might give consideration to surgery wherein the ductal systems of both breasts are excised. This procedure is seldom necessary for this condition. When a woman whose breasts secrete milk approaches menopause, the secretion will stop spontaneously.

Pus. The secretion of pus indicates the presence of an underlying infection. The pus should be cultured and antibiotic sensitivity tests conducted. If the discharge continues despite appropriate antibiotic medication, then incision and drainage of the infection must be carried out.

Watery, straw-colored, pinkish, or bloody discharges from the nipple command careful investigation to discover the underlying breast disorder. Statistics * show that abnormal nipple discharge of one of the above types occurs in approximately 8 percent of those patients who require surgery for a benign or malignant lesion of the breast. In some 1,868 consecutive cases of benign and malignant breast disease, nipple discharge occurred in 152 cases, but cancer was associated with nipple discharge in only 19,

---

* H. P. Leis, Jr., and S. Pilnick, writing in *Hospital Medicine,* November 1970.

or 1 percent, of all cases. However, it was an accompaniment of cancer in almost 4 percent of the 504 cancer cases in the group.

The most common cause for the nipple discharge described above is an *intraductal papilloma,* or warty growth arising from one of the major ducts leading to the nipple. The second most common cause is *cystic disease* of the breast. The third most common lesion leading to nipple discharge is *ectasia.* These conditions are dealt with elsewhere in this book and their characteristics will not be repeated here.

Bloody discharge from the nipple is noted occasionally among pregnant women. This is a functional phenomenon and is not a sign of breast disease.

A word should be said about cytological examination of material discharged from the nipple. This procedure involves smearing some of the discharge onto a glass slide, staining it, and examining its cells under a microscope. Diagnosis of breast lesions through study of cells in the nipple discharge requires great expertise by the pathologist or cytologist. Although there are some pathology departments that claim an 80 percent accurate diagnostic rate, most hospitals are not so fortunate in this regard. Suspicious discharges should be examined in all instances and the surgeon should rely on a *positive* finding. In other words, if a smear from a nipple discharge shows malignant cells, it has great significance. However, the absence of malignant cells is no proof that the patient is free of cancer, and it would indicate further need of examination.

Even when no visible discharge is present, in a few clinics throughout the country techniques have evolved wherein cells are suctioned from the ducts of the nipple. A tiny catheter is inserted into the major duct of the nipple, a small amount of liquid is injected and then retrieved by gentle suction. Cells so obtained are submitted to cytological examination under a microscope.

Questions and Answers

Do women ever have unequal-sized nipples?
Yes, but it is not nearly as common as unequal-sized breasts.

Can anything be done to make the nipples more equal in size?
This is seldom indicated as it may cause deformity of both nipples.

Why is it that some women always seem to have flat, flaccid nipples?
This is not so. They contract and become erect during cold weather or on stimulation.

Why is it that nursing a baby does not cause sexual stimulation?
Similar stimuli may evoke various reactions, according to the emotional attitude of the individual. The mother does get a sensuous pleasure from nursing, but it differs from that which she experiences with her mate.

Do women continue to receive erotic sensations from stimulation of the nipples even though they have gone through change of life?
Yes. Menopause has little to do with a woman's sexual response.

At what age do women develop breast discharge?
Most discharges of the breast occur in women prior to the menopause. When breast discharge takes place in women past the menopause it is more significant because it might indicate the presence of a malignant tumor.

At what other times in life do women ever develop a nipple discharge that is not indicative of disease?
1. Some young women may have a slight clear or straw-colored discharge from the nipple associated with menstruation.
2. Women who are at menopause may accidentally discover that when they squeeze their nipple there will be a small amount of discharge.
Neither of these conditions indicates the presence of breast disease, nor is any therapy needed to overcome it.

Will overactive stimulation of the breasts cause a discharge?

There might be a very slight colorless discharge of fluid from the nipple of the breast following overly vigorous breast stimulation, but this is not significant.

What is the significance of excretion of greenish, brownish, or reddish material from the nipple?

It is more likely to indicate the presence of an intraductal papilloma, but other conditions, enumerated in this chapter, must also be considered as possibilities.

Is there a great difference between the discharge of greenish-colored, brownish-colored, or bloody discharge from the breasts?

No. The greenish and brownish discharge from the breasts merely indicates that there is a small quantity of blood being secreted from the papilloma within the breast and this blood changes in color from green to brown as it remains within the ducts. When the discharge is frankly bloody in character, it indicates that more bleeding is taking place and is being discharged more rapidly from the breast.

Should a woman wait after noting a greenish, brownish, or bloody discharge from the nipple before she consults a physician?

Such a discharge is an indication for an early medical consultation.

Is it frequent that a woman has discharge from her breast and doesn't notice it?

Unless there is a very slight amount of colorless discharge from the breast it will usually be noticed when a woman takes off her brassiere or nightgown.

Do women have pain when they have discharge from their nipples?
No.

Will the taking of oral contraceptives cause discharge from the nipples?

Some women who have taken oral contraceptives for a long period of time may develop a clear or milky discharge from the nipples. It usually occurs from both breasts and does not contain blood. It has no significance and can be ignored.

Is it more urgent to operate on an older woman who has discharge from her breasts?

Yes, especially when the discharge is bloody in nature. Women past the menopause who have bloody discharge from the nipples may have actively growing intraductal papillomas. Because these conditions are precancerous, it is essential that they be removed early in their development.

Do intraductal papillomas of the breast ever become cancerous?

On occasion, yes. This is one of the few truly precancerous lesions of the breast.

25 BENIGN SOLID TUMORS AND LESIONS OF THE BREAST

As we have seen—and contrary to common belief—most lumps or lesions in the breast are benign. The family physician who first examines the patient with a breast lesion will encounter a benign condition approximately 90 percent of the time.

The most commonly encountered benign lesions of the breast, exclusive of cysts and cystic disease (see following chapter), are the following:

1. *Fibroadenomas* (adenofibromas) are true tumors, seen most often in young women between fifteen and thirty-five years of age. They vary in size from that of a pea to an orange. Usually they occur as single tumors, but occasionally two or more may be present at the same time.

Fibroadenomas, as the name suggests, are composed of both fibrous and gland tissues. They rarely present a diagnostic problem because of their characteristic firm, solid, round feel to the touch. The tumors are freely movable within the breast, are surrounded by a sharply outlined border, and are nontender. They do not attach themselves to the overlying skin of the breast.

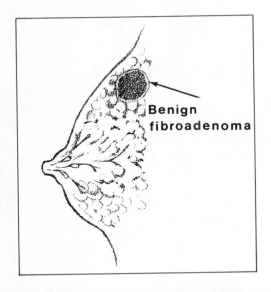

Benign
fibroadenoma

Benign tumors located far from the center of the breast must be removed through small incisions directly over the lump. The scar will fade in time.

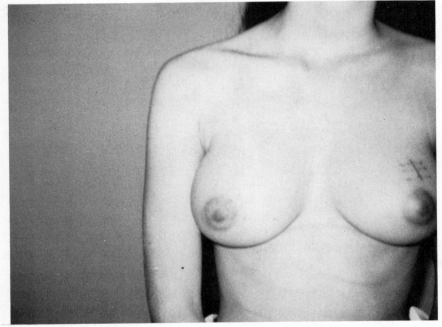

The cause of fibroadenomas is obscure, but they are not thought to be related to hormonal upset, as the glandular function in patients with these tumors is usually normal.

The diagnosis of fibroadenoma is so simple that it is seldom necessary to send these patients for mammography or thermography, nor is needle biopsy indicated.

Treatment for fibroadenoma is surgical removal. The operation takes only a few minutes to perform as the tumor shells out readily because of its well-defined capsule. The patient can leave the hospital within one to three days after surgery, and can return to work or to her household duties after a few days' time, if she so desires. This of course excludes the extraordinary number of emotional side effects from even the most minor breast surgery, including that of a letdown feeling, headache, dizziness, lack of appetite, and depression. Emotional instability may persist for several weeks.

Every once in a while a physician finds a fibroadenoma in an older woman. If he takes a careful history, he will discover that the lump had been present for many years and that the patient had never bothered to undergo a breast examination. In these cases, the diagnosis of malignancy comes to mind because of the patient's age, and the patient is in most instances referred for mammography. If the lump has been in existence for many years, the mammogram may show a calcium deposit but it is not the type seen in cancer.

Fibroadenomas, in all probability, do not become malignant, but in a few instances cancers have been discovered growing within the capsule of fibroadenomas. One may ask, "Why, if fibroadenomas do not become malignant, is it necessary to remove them?" The answer is that fibroadenomas tend to grow to large size and may deform the breast. Secondly, unless a tumor is removed, one cannot be absolutely certain that it is benign.

2. *Lipoma* is a frequently encountered benign tumor in the breast. Lipomas are composed of fat tissues that are rather well encapsulated and thus easily distinguished from the surrounding normal breast. They cannot be seen on mammography nor do they appear as "hot" areas on thermography. However, they represent no diagnostic problem. Lipomas occur more often in stout than thin women. They are painless.

Lipomas of the breast are treated in the same manner as lipomas anywhere else in the body. They can be left alone, as they rarely undergo cancerous degeneration. Their removal is recommended, however, whenever there is the slightest doubt as to diagnosis or when the tumor is large and disfigures breast contours; also when the tumor begins to grow rapidly.

As with all benign breast lesions, surgery is a simple matter requiring no more than two to three days' hospitalization.

3. *Intraductal papilloma, intraductal hyperplasia,* and *intraductal papillomatosis.* We have looked at these earlier, briefly. An intraductal papilloma is a warty growth within one of the ducts of the breast; intraductal hyperplasia is an overgrowth of the cells lining the ducts; intraductal papillomatosis is a condition similar to intraductal papilloma but it involves most of the ducts within the breast. These lesions are characterized by a nipple discharge, which may be colorless, yellowish, greenish, or bloody. Often there is no palpable lump, the first sign of the condition being a stain in a brassiere or on night clothes.

A single intraductal papilloma is sometimes accompanied by a small, pea-sized, nontender lump beneath the nipple. If no lump is present, the examining surgeon can frequently locate the site of the lesion by gently pressing various points about the circumference of the nipple. The lesion is located beneath the point at which the pressure evokes a discharge from the nipple. Intraductal hyperplasia is not accompanied by a localized tumor but the diagnosis of intraductal hyperplasia can be suspected because of nipple discharge.

In intraductal papillomatosis, pressure at several points may express discharge from the nipple. Palpable masses are unusual in this condition, the diagnosis depending on the nipple discharge.

Neither mammography nor thermography is significantly diagnostic in these conditions, although dilated ducts are sometimes observed.

After obtaining a drop or two of the secretions from the nipple—the amount seldom exceeds a few drops—the surgeon will spread it out on a glass slide and forward it to the pathologist for microscopic examination. Unfortunately, the results of these examinations are not often rewarding. Secretions from the nipple yield much less information than the Pap smears taken from the cervix and vagina.

Although benign, intraductal papilloma, hyperplasia, and papillomatosis are considered by many physicians to be truly precancerous lesions. If they go untreated, there is always the possibility that the cells within the ducts will undergo cancerous changes. For this reason, surgery is often indicated for these conditions. The operation involves a semicircular incision (periareolar) around that part of the nipple where it joins the surrounding skin of the breast. The incision measures one to two inches in length. The nipple is reflected, thus exposing the ducts that empty into it. If the lesion is a single intraductal papilloma, the surgeon will note a single dilated duct. He will dissect out this duct, open it, and locate the tiny warty growth. These growths vary in size from that of a caraway seed to a small pea. The duct is excised from beneath the nipple down into the breast structure to a point beyond the papilloma. Before replacing the nipple to its normal position and suturing it back to its surrounding skin, the surgeon makes sure that no other ducts are dilated or contain papillomas. If other ducts are dilated, it indicates that the condition probably involves the entire ductal system of the breast. In this event, the entire ductal system should be excised. The severed edges of breast tissue would be sutured after removing the ducts and the nipple stitched back into place. No deformity results from this operation.

Women with intraductal lesions should be advised beforehand that they might be faced with a slightly longer hospital stay until a final diagnosis is forthcoming. The reason is that frozen-section examinations of intraductal lesions are notoriously difficult to interpret, as many sections must be cut to be absolutely certain that malignant changes have not taken place.

If malignant changes are found, which occurs only occasionally, they often are confined to the ducts and the tissues immediately surrounding the ducts. This type of cancer not infrequently lends itself to simple mastectomy and affords the patient an excellent chance for permanent cure.

Any woman who has undergone excision of one intraductal papilloma is a candidate for a similar lesion in the same or opposite breast. She should therefore undergo breast examination at least three times a year.

4. *Fibrosis* of the breast means replacement of glandular tissue by inert fibrous tissues. This is a natural process which takes place in every breast as one ages. However, the process may be quite uneven in that it affects certain portions of the breast much more than others. As a result, a patch of fibrosis surrounded by normal glandular tissue may give the impression of a tumor mass. Mammography and thermography may not contribute much information in these cases because they are almost always negative. As I have mentioned before, a negative mammogram or thermogram is

not proof that a lesion is benign. Therefore, in cases of fibrosis accompanied by a dominant lump, excisional biopsy is indicated, especially since women with this condition are in the cancer-bearing age group. The frozen-section examination in these cases will invariably reveal the nature of the pathology, thus permitting a short hospitalization.

5. *Sclerosing adenosis* is a benign lesion seen in women during the child-bearing period of their lives. Its cause is obscure, and abnormal glandular function is not an accompanying feature of the disease. Adenosis means overgrowth of the glandular structure of the breast to such an extent that the gland tissues replace some of the surrounding connective tissues. This process stimulates a response from the surrounding tissues in which ensues a fibrous reaction to choke off, or sclerose, the glandular overgrowth. Thus, the term sclerosing adenosis.

The process may proceed within the breast without ever forming a dominant lump, in which event the condition never comes to the attention of a physician. It is only when a dominant tumor mass appears that surgical excision is recommended.

Sclerosing adenosis cannot usually be diagnosed specifically on manual examination and it sometimes feels very much like cancer. Mammography and thermography are negative in this condition but, as stated before, this fact should not contraindicate operative investigation.

Although sclerosing adenosis does not turn into cancer, surgical removal of the localized area is carried out to make certain of the diagnosis. Recovery is rapid, as with other benign lesions. Despite the removal of one area of adenosis, other areas of the breast may at some future time develop sclerosing adenosis and they, too, should be biopsied. Fortunately, the tendency to form these tumors ends with menopause.

6. *Cystosarcoma phyllodes* is a tumor composed of both glandular and fibrous tissues. One of its outstanding characteristics is that it can grow to tremendous size. A fourteen-year-old patient of mine had a lump smaller than a dime that grew to the size of a grapefruit within a period of eight months.

Cystosarcoma phyllodes affects mainly younger women who, because of the rapid rate of growth of the tumors, become very alarmed. Whereas the condition is considered to be benign, there are cases on record wherein the tumor either recurred locally after removal or metastasized, that is, spread to distant organs. Wide surgical removal of these tumors is recommended, and if any microscopic evidence of malignancy is found, breast removal is indicated. Fortunately, these tumors are uncommon, and malignant degeneration is rare.

7. *Ectasia*, or more precisely, *mammary duct ectasia*, is a condition characterized by marked dilatation of the ducts of the breast. The ducts become enlarged and distended with debris from gland and duct cells that have disintegrated. As a result, a fatty, yellowish green or brownish semisolid substance fills the ducts. In general, the process affects all the ducts but it may be more prominent in one area than another. Ectasia is frequently associated with cystic formation as the ducts distend and become round. Some of the ducts may become inflamed as a result of ectasia and they rupture, allowing for the escape of the semisolid excretion into surrounding breast tissue. The invaded breast tissue becomes inflamed, and as the inflammation subsides calcium deposits may form, eventually leading to considerable breast destruction and deformity.

Ectasia has its onset during the forties and may continue past menopause. Usually, the process affects both breasts and involves, to a lesser or greater extent, the entire ductal system.

Surgery for ectasia can be quite challenging as so much tissue is involved that total removal of the diseased area would require subcutaneous mastectomy (see Subcutaneous Mastectomy). Short of that procedure, the entire ductal system of the breast and all cysts that have formed from the ducts must be removed. This may leave considerable deformity that can be minimized only by careful breast reconstruction. The immediate postoperative appearance may not be good, though normal breast contours tend to return after several months' time.

Ectasia is not a very common condition. It does not lead to cancer.

8. *Lobular neoplasia* is a precancerous condition sometimes encountered accidentally when operating for an unrelated breast lesion. It has also been termed *cancer in situ*, a form of malignancy that has not yet become invasive.

Lobular neoplasia is a microscopic diagnosis, made only when the pathologist sees gland and duct structures that appear to be in the process of becoming cancerous. The neoplasia may exist in several widely separated places in a breast. One of the disturbing things about this disorder is that it produces no dominant lump. Its discovery, therefore, is usually accidental.

Lobular neoplasia occurs in women during their thirties or forties, while they are still having menstrual periods. It may develop into true cancer, or it may disappear completely with the onset of menopause.

Lobular neoplasia constitutes a most powerful argument in favor of removing the entire breast whenever a cancer exists, no matter how small it may be or no matter where it is located in the breast: a cancerous lump may be limited to only one site, but many other areas of the same breast may be involved in lobular neoplasia. If the surgeon in such a case performs merely a "lumpectomy," or a partial mastectomy, he may leave behind a potentially cancerous area in another part of the breast.

The safest procedure to recommend to a patient with lobular neoplasia is that she undergo subcutaneous mastectomy with simultaneous or delayed insertion of a plastic implant to restore breast contour. Only in this way can subsequent cancer be avoided in many of these patients.

9. *Fat necrosis* is a condition resulting from destruction of fat cells due to a direct injury, to rapid weight loss, or to changes brought about by aging. When the fat tissue of the breast dies, it is frequently replaced by fibrous tissue, sometimes accompanied by deposits of calcium. This gives that area of the breast a firm, hard, irregular feel to the touch, not unlike the feel of a cancer. Mammography may be helpful since calcium deposits in cancer have a different appearance from those in fat necrosis. However, to be as safe as possible, surgery, with local removal of the lesion and its immediate examination under the microscope, is recommended.

10. *Moles* (*nevi*). The breast is a common site for the location of a mole. Moles are not actual breast tumors, but their surgical removal is indicated if they grow, change in color, bleed, or are subject to repeated irritation from a brassiere.

11. *Breast hypertrophy,* the *adolescent nodule, gynecomastia,* and *hematoma* are discussed elsewhere in this book and will therefore not be dealt with here.

Questions and Answers

Does surgical removal of a benign tumor ever stir up the breast so that it develops a cancer?

No. There was a time several decades ago when folklore had it that operating would stir up a cancer. This is completely untrue.

Can a surgeon tell, before an operation, whether a lump is benign?

In the great majority of cases the surgeon *can* make a correct diagnosis. However, this is not good enough—100 percent accuracy must be the goal. Only after the lump has been removed and a section carefully examined under a microscope—and only then—can a diagnosis be made with complete certainty.

What kind of operation is usually done to remove a benign tumor?

Simple removal of a lump through an incision is usually all that is required. The incision may vary from one to three inches in length, depending on the size of the underlying lump.

How long a hospital stay is necessary after removal of a benign lump?

If a simple excision of a mass has been performed, the patient may be released within one to three days postoperatively. If a drain has been inserted into the depths of the wound, the surgeon may ask the patient to stay an additional day or two until the drain has been removed.

What differentiates a cyst from a fibroadenoma?

A fibroadenoma tends to be firmer and to be more movable within the substance of the breast than a cyst. Also, fibroadenomas are much more frequently seen in women under 35 years of age, whereas cysts are more common over 35 years of age. Mammography can frequently distinguish a solid tumor from a fluid-containing cyst.

Can a surgeon distinguish between a benign and malignant tumor by examining a breast with his hand?

Usually. Nevertheless, a microscopic examination is more accurate because no matter how great the diagnostic ability of the surgeon, he can make mistakes on examining a breast.

What are the features that distinguish a benign tumor from a cancer?

Most benign tumors are rather freely movable within the breast substance, they are rounded in shape, and are not attached to the overlying skin; cancers tend to be irregular and fixed in position within the breast and are frequently attached to the undersurface of the skin.

Can a surgeon diagnose a specific type of benign tumor by breast examination?

Fibroadenomas can often be distinguished from an area of fat necrosis, from an intraductal papilloma, and from a lipoma. However, it may not be easy to tell a fibroadenoma from a cystosarcoma phyllodes or from an area of sclerosing adenosis.

What harm can come from observing a supposed benign lump within a breast?

If the examining surgeon happens to be wrong in his diagnosis, it will permit time for the cancer to spread to the glands beneath the armpit. It is far better to have a harmless lesion removed than to allow a cancer to go untreated for a period of weeks or months.

Do benign tumors respond to X-ray or cobalt treatment?
No.

Will benign conditions ever respond to hormone therapy?

Certain breasts that are involved in chronic cystic disease may respond to hormone therapy, but most solid tumors are unaffected by this form of treatment.

How soon after a lump have been found should surgery be performed?

As soon as a lump has been discovered, arrangements should be made for its removal, that is, within a period of two to three weeks.

Should a woman allow herself to become pregnant after removal of a benign tumor of the breast?

Yes, it is perfectly permissible.

Can a woman resume intercourse soon after being discharged for the removal of a benign condition?

Yes, the only precaution is that the breast that has been operated on not be hurt during the act of intercourse.

Is the operation for removal of a benign tumor painful?

No. Pain in the wound area and pain in the remainder of the breast may occur postoperatively if there has been seepage of blood into the depths of the wound. It should be remembered that even in the removal of benign tumors, a sizable amount of breast tissue has been removed. The space left behind often contains serum or blood. A collection of serum or blood in the depths of a breast wound is not at all uncommon, and this collection may produce pain.

When does the surgeon place a drain in a wound?
When he expects a large collection of serum or blood to follow the removal of a lump. The larger the lump, the more likely will this be.

Is it ever necessary for a surgeon to remove the serum or blood that collects in the depths of a breast wound?
Yes. In some instances, the serum or blood will ooze spontaneously in between the sutures of such an incision; in other cases, the surgeon may place an instrument into the depths of the wound to let out the collected serum or blood, or he may remove it with a needle and syringe.

Is healing delayed by the accumulation of serum or blood in the depths of a breast wound?
Yes. A wound that collects a large amount of serum or blood may take two to three weeks before it has completely healed.

How soon after an operation for a benign breast tumor can one bathe?
As soon as the wound has healed.

Do benign breast tumors tend to be inherited?
There is no proof that benign breast tumors are inherited.

26 CYSTIC DISEASE OF THE BREAST

Cystic disease is the most common disorder of the female breast. Though statistics differ from one reporter to another, it is safe to conjecture that 1 out of 6 women between the age of 35 and 50 years has some form of this disease.

There have been several names given to this condition, namely *fibrocystic disease, chronic cystic mastitis, chronic cystic disease, Schimmelbusch's disease, lumpy breasts, shoddy breasts,* and others. No matter what name is used, the pathological findings in the disorder are the same. True cystic disease must show cysts, even if they are microscopic in size. In these cases, the diagnosis is made only on examination of breast tissue by the pathologist. Accompanying the formation of the cysts, there is usually overgrowth of the cells lining the cysts and their surrounding ducts, and an increase in the adjacent fibrous tissues. Thus, the name *fibrocystic disease.*

The importance of cystic disease cannot be overemphasized as it is calculated that cancer is three times more apt to occur in a breast affected by the condition.

The exact cause of cystic disease is not known, but women with the disorder are in the estrogen-producing years of life. Cysts also are frequently seen in women who regularly take large doses of estrogen. It is more probable that the estrogen stimulates growth of preexisting cysts rather than initiating the disease in a normal breast. The influence of estrogen is further evidenced by the fact that cystic disease tends to dis-

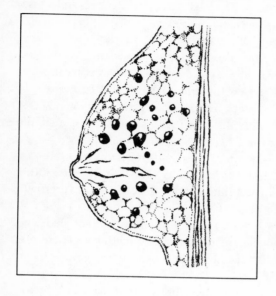

Cystic disease is characterized by the formation of innumerable small and large cysts, usually located throughout the breast.

appear with the onset of menopause, and has usually disappeared completely by the end of the menopausal years.

Cystic disease may involve every portion of both breasts or it may be limited to small areas in one or both breasts. In mild forms of the disorder, lumps may not be felt at all; in moderate cystic disease, the breasts may feel shoddy or lumpy throughout, without the formation of a dominant lump or lumps; in advanced stages, one or more isolated cysts, small or large, can be felt. Some cysts can grow larger than a hen's egg.

The signs of cystic disease can fluctuate markedly, depending on the time of month that the patient is examined. Generally, because of the swelling of the breasts for the few days prior to the onset of menstruation, if the breasts are felt then, they may reveal a definite cyst. But on re-examination in the intermenstrual period, the cyst may seem to have disappeared. Most surgeons therefore request that their patients be checked at various times during the menstrual cycle.

Some women have no symptoms from cystic disease whereas others suffer considerable pain in the breasts, especially during the premenstrual period. When a cyst grows rapidly, its walls become distended and tense, resulting in pain and marked tenderness.

Relatively little permanent help can be given to those who suffer periodic breast pain due to cystic disease. Some physicians recommend diuretic drugs to be taken during the few days prior to menstruation in the hope that dehydration will lessen the engorgement and tenderness of the breasts. But this form of therapy is too drastic to recommend as a routine procedure. A much better medication for this condition is a simple pain-relieving drug such as aspirin.

Some of the cysts are thin walled, giving a bluish color as one approaches them at operation. These are known as blue-domed cysts. Other cysts are very thick walled, and their lining shows a heaped-up overgrowth of cells.

Since cystic disease is in a sense a metabolic condition associated with a hormone imbalance, it cannot be cured by surgical methods. Therefore, surgery is carried out mainly for diagnostic purposes or to remove a cyst that is causing pain.

We have seen that when a woman develops a large mass in a breast, it is not always possible to distinguish whether the lesion is a cyst or a solid tumor, and that mammography may not reveal the diagnosis, either. To obtain a broader view of the practice of American surgeons in the treatment of cysts, I polled various professors of surgery at medical colleges throughout the country. Of 39 who replied, only 13, or 33⅓ percent, thought that aspiration (inserting a needle and extracting the fluid for examination) was an adequate method of investigating and treating a breast with a definable lump caused by a cyst. The other 26 surgeons believed, as do I, that a woman with cystic disease associated with a dominant lump should be subjected to an operation for removal of the cyst. If she comes from a breast cancer family, it is especially important that she undergo at least one cyst removal. It was the contention of the various professors that the exact nature of a particular patient's disease process can best be determined after gross and microscopic examination of the cyst *and the surrounding tissues and ducts.* Also, these surgeons contend that not infrequently a malignant growth is found accompanying a cyst.

Over the years I have encountered quite a few cases in which a malignancy has been discovered in close proximity to a cyst. In addition,

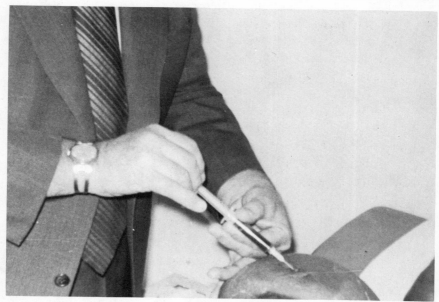

Single, large cysts can sometimes be treated by aspiration only. It is a relatively painless office procedure.

I have had many cases in which the lining of a cyst, and the lining of the ducts surrounding the cyst, has shown marked overgrowth (hyperplasia) of its cells. As this pathology may be a forerunner of cancer, it is important to have this information. Such information cannot be obtained by mere aspiration of the cyst, as microscopic examination of cyst fluid is notoriously unrewarding in the majority of cases. Moreover, aspiration of fluid from a cyst cannot give one an idea of the nature of a disease process that might be progressing in the wall of, or in the tissues surrounding the cyst. In this connection, it might be interesting to cite the following case:

A 42-year-old female presented herself with a large cyst in her left breast. When she was informed that aspiration was to be performed, she refused, stating that her gynecologist had attempted aspiration but could not obtain any fluid. She wanted the lump out of her breast, she said. The cyst was removed, and the pathologist reported a thick-walled cyst, surrounded by ducts showing marked overgrowth (ductal hyperplasia with papillomatosis) of their lining cells. He appended a note to his report stating: "Patient should be followed up carefully because of the florid duct hyperplasia."

During the next 5 years, the patient formed 4 more cysts, and each time she refused aspiration and insisted on their surgical removal. The cysts varied in size from 1 to 2 inches in diameter. Each time, the tissue surrounding the cysts showed marked overgrowth of the cells lining the ducts.

Seven years after the appearance of her first cyst, this patient underwent radical mastectomy for a cancer that was located about $1\frac{1}{2}$ inches from the incision for removal of her original cyst.

This does not imply that one of the patient's cysts eventually became malignant. Rather, the point is that women with cystic disease and accompanying duct disease, a common combination, have breasts that are prone to cancer. They must therefore be examined at least every few months until menopause has taken place and the tendency to form cysts has subsided.

In general, those surgeons who routinely aspirate rather than excise cysts agree that if fluid collects again after aspiration, it is wise to remove the cyst. A cyst that fills up again with fluid may have a cancer growing from the membrane lining its wall. Fortunately, these cases constitute a minority.

The two other types of cysts seen in breasts which are not part of the condition we have labelled *cystic disease* are:

1. *Galactoceles* (milk cysts) are caused by the blockage of a milk duct. It is seen in women who have recently borne children. A galactocele can be aspirated in an attempt to avoid surgery, but in some cases they fill up again. When this happens the cyst should be removed surgically. It is a simple operation, followed by rapid recovery.

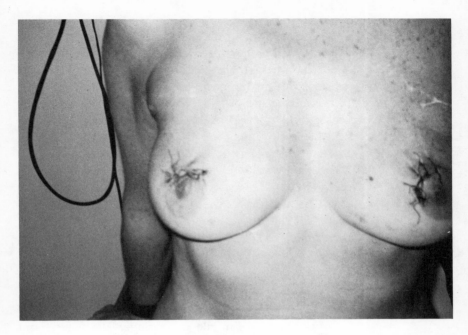

Incisions for removal of many large cysts of both breasts are made above the nipples. Seen here are the incisions with the stitches in place and one month later. The scars will eventually fade.

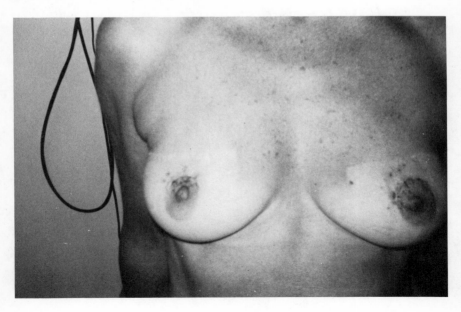

2. *Sebaceous cysts* have a predilection for the skin of the breasts and for the cleavage area between the breasts. This type of cyst results from the blockage of the skin opening of an oil (sebaceous) gland.

Sebaceous cysts can be readily excised under local anesthesia. If they are not removed, they tend to grow large and to become infected. Once infection has set in, they can only be incised, resulting in a wound that may drain for several weeks. Then, when the infection has subsided completely, it will be necessary to excise the cyst. To avoid double surgery, it is therefore best to remove these lesions before they become infected.

Questions and Answers

What is the treatment for cystic disease?
1. Aspiration of the cyst with needle and syringe. The fluid is sent to the laboratory and examined for malignant cells.
2. Surgical removal of the cyst.

Should cysts be aspirated with a needle or removed surgically?
There are cases in which one or the other form of treatment is applicable. Surgical removal of a cyst gives much valuable additional information concerning the pathology of breast tissue surrounding the cyst. Thus, it is perhaps best to undergo surgery for the first definite cyst that forms, and to have aspiration for subsequent cysts. Of course, if a cyst fills up again after aspiration, or if suspicious cells are seen on examination of the aspirated fluid, the cyst should be removed surgically.

Can surgery cure cystic disease?
No.

Is it painful to aspirate a cyst?
No. The surgeon will usually give a drop or two of Novocain in the skin and will insert the aspirating needle in the anesthetized area. There is remarkably little pain from breast aspiration even when local anesthesia is not given.

Can fluid be removed from every cyst?

No. Sometimes, the breast contains a very thick tan or brownish substance that will not come through the aspirating needle. These cysts are frequently found in association with a condition known as ectasia, wherein the milk ducts are widely dilated and thickened.

Can one tell on aspiration whether a cyst will form again or not?

No. This will depend greatly on the character of the lining membrane of the cyst and whether there is diffuse pathology associated with the cyst. Some cysts occur in breasts that show evidence of great cellular activity, and if this is so, recurrence of cysts is very likely.

Does aspiration of a cyst stimulate it to fill up again?
No.

Will aspiration of a cyst stimulate a tumor to grow within the breast?
No.

Will needling a lump in the breast, on the erroneous assumption that it contains a cyst, cause the spread of tumor cells?

Usually, a surgeon can distinguish between a cyst and solid tumor, so that he rarely aspirates a tumor by mistake. However, even if he does, he will not spread the tumor as there will be ample time for him to arrange for its surgical removal before a spread can take place.

Can a woman who has had a cyst removed be permitted to nurse a baby?

Yes. The existence of such a lesion has no bearing whatever on nursing.

Is a woman who has had cystic disease during her premenopausal years more likely to develop a cyst after menopause, if she takes estrogens?
Yes.

27 SUBCUTANEOUS MASTECTOMY

Subcutaneous mastectomy is an operative procedure in which most of the breast tissue is removed, but the overlying nipple and surrounding skin, with its attached fat, is undisturbed. The primary objective of this operation is to excise as much gland tissue as possible, usually more than 95 percent, while retaining the superficial covering of the breast. If the patient is full breasted, subcutaneous mastectomy often results in an unattractive, empty sac on the chest wall. In order to overcome this appearance, a plastic operation to excise redundant tissues may be carried out along with the subcutaneous mastectomy, or a plastic silastic bag may be inserted to restore normal contours. If the breast is small to begin with, subcutaneous mastectomy may not alter contours to any significant extent.

To date, subcutaneous mastectomy is not a very widely employed operation in the treatment of breast disease. As we have seen, cancer is treated by total breast removal whereas benign lesions are locally excised. However, it is realized more clearly each year that certain benign conditions, such as cystic disease, intraductal overgrowths, and lobular neoplasia, predispose toward eventual cancer. As a consequence, subcutaneous mastectomy is being considered as a prophylactic cancer prevention operation. Although it may appear to be drastic surgery to recommend for a patient with a noncancerous breast disorder, there is a rather large group of women who would benefit greatly from its performance. The main candidates are:

1. Patients with a strong history of breast cancer in the family who have multiple cysts throughout both their breasts, and although they have undergone repeated aspiration and local cyst removals, continue to form new cysts.

People in this category are three times more likely to develop breast cancer than women without a familial history of breast cancer and without cystic disease.

2. Patients with a strong history of breast cancer in the family who have intraductal hyperplasia (overgrowth of the cells lining the ducts) or intraductal papillomas (warty growths) who, despite surgical removal of these lesions, continue to form new areas of hyperplasia or papillomas.

This group of individuals is also three times more prone to develop breast cancer than those not in this category.

3. Patients who have had one breast removed because of cancer and whose other breast is the seat either of cystic disease or intraductal pathology such as hyperplasia or papillomas.

A woman who has had one breast involved in cancer is more prone than others to develop a malignancy within the opposite breast, especially if the remaining breast is affected by intraductal pathology or cystic disease.

4. Patients who have been found to have areas of lobular neoplasia in their breasts. This condition is usually found accidentally when operating on the breast for some other lesion. Lobular neoplasia is thought to be a definitely precancerous condition, much like the "cancer in situ" seen in the cervix. Happily, it is not a commonly encountered disorder.

Subcutaneous mastectomy is not complicated to perform. A horizontal crescentic incision approximately 4 inches long is made in the fold beneath the breast (the inframammary crease). There is a rather bloodless plane between the chest wall and the overlying breast, making it a simple matter to dissect away the gland tissues. The surgeon next separates the breast tissue from the overlying subcutaneous tissues and skin and, when the dissection is completed, he can remove almost the entire gland in one piece. A small amount of breast tissue is usually left behind directly beneath the nipple. The nipple and the skin of the breast are nourished by the blood vessels that travel through the fatty subcutaneous tissues.

On completing the subcutaneous mastectomy a decision is made whether to insert a plastic implant to restore normal contours, whether to reduce the size of the "breast sac" by excising redundant skin, or whether to defer either of these procedures until several weeks later. However, when a plastic implant is employed there can be complications:

1. Because thin women usually have little fat beneath the skin of their breasts, the plastic implant may cause erosion (ulceration) of the overlying skin, with eventual infection and rejection of the implant.

2. Technical errors in carrying out the operation in any woman may deprive the overlying skin of essential blood supply, again resulting in erosion and ultimate rejection of the implant.

3. Infection occurs in a small but definite number of patients who undergo this procedure. Infection surrounding the implant almost always leads to its rejection and eventual extrusion.

4. If bleeding in the depths of the wound has not been controlled absolutely, infection may set in and the implant will be rejected.

5. Some patients are extremely dissatisfied with the final cosmetic result after subcutaneous mastectomy and the employment of an implant. This group is small, but little can be done for them except to remove the implant. They are seldom willing to submit to a secondary operation with insertion of a new implant.

On the positive side, however, through subcutaneous mastectomy, the patient is relieved of a good deal of the fear that she will subsequently develop a breast cancer, and she willingly accepts in its stead the possible cosmetic disfigurement which sometimes follows this operation.

Questions and Answers

Are the scars very disfiguring following subcutaneous mastectomy?
No, they are made beneath the breast in the inframammary crease.

What types of implants are used after removing the breast tissue?
One of two types, a silastic bag into which ordinary saline (salt solution) is injected, according to the size of the breast one wants to attain; or a silastic bag of fixed size containing a silicone gel.

Is it ever possible to reinsert a breast implant if it has once been removed for infection?
Yes, but several months' time must elapse before this should be attempted.

Are the chances greater for rejection to take place again, if it has once taken place?
Yes.

Are implants always inserted after performing a subcutaneous mastectomy?
No. Some women show little interest in the cosmetic result of the procedure. Their main aim is to rid themselves of the danger of breast cancer.

Is it feasible to perform the subcutaneous mastectomy at one time, and the insertion of the plastic implant at a later date?
Yes. Some surgeons prefer to do it this way.

Can a woman who has decided against a plastic implant change her mind and have the operation done several weeks or months after the subcutaneous mastectomy?
Yes, but it is somewhat more difficult to perform and the ultimate results are not quite as good.

28 CANCER OF THE BREAST

Cancer of the breast is one of the world's greatest unconquered killers. It is a mean, nasty, capricious, unpredictable disease that grows silently and without symptoms until, in far too many cases, it has spread beyond cure by the time it is discovered. As a result, half the women who develop breast cancer succumb to it within ten years. The disease *demands* that the medical profession come up with new ways to diagnose it before there has been any spread. If this could be accomplished, over 85 to 90 percent of those afflicted could be cured.

Here are some significant statistics:

1. According to the last United States Bureau of the Census figures, there are now 60 million females 25 years of age or older in our country.

2. The average American female 25 years of age who is presently in good health has a life expectancy of 51 more years, according to the Metropolitan Life Insurance Company's Life Expectancy Tables.

3. Ninety thousand new cases of breast cancer develop each year in the United States, according to the American Cancer Society.

4. With 90,000 new cases of breast cancer appearing each year and with our adult females living for 51 more years, it

is probable that 4,590,000 of the 60,000,000 will one day develop breast cancer.

5. In a monumental statistical and epidemiological study conducted under the auspices of the American Cancer Society,* involving many thousands of cases, it has been shown that 61 percent of all breast cancers treated by standard methods survive for 5 years, 50 percent survive for 10 years, and 42 percent survive for 20 years. This study includes cases in all stages of development, including those in which the tumor has spread to the nodes in the armpit. When seen and treated before spread of the disease to the lymph nodes in the armpit, and when subjected to the so-called "radical" mastectomy, 80 to 85 percent of the patients survive for 5 or more years.

The unfortunate part of statistics in breast cancer is that they show too little improvement in survival rates over the past 50 years. The question arises over and over again in the minds of those who are interested in this subject whether the failure to obtain greater improvement in survival rates is caused by too late detection of disease, by inadequate surgery, the wrong type of surgery, surgery performed too late in the course of the disease, or to utilizing surgery rather than some other modality as the main form of treatment. There is general agreement that surgery is *not* a fundamental form of therapy. Surgery is symptomatic treatment; it cuts out a tumor that has already formed, and all one can do is to hope that the entire tumor has been removed at a point before it has spread beyond the reach of the scalpel. Too often, this is not the case. Improvement in surgical cures must therefore depend greatly on earlier detection of the breast cancer.

It is also agreed generally that irradiation, chemotherapy, hormone therapy, and surgery to eliminate possible harmful hormone secretions are mainly adjunct, palliative forms of therapy that attempt to prolong the life of one whose cancer has spread beyond ultimate control. However, recent work with new anticancer chemicals would seem to indicate that their use postoperatively may actually destroy and prevent the growth of cancer cells that have spread from the breast to distant areas of the body.

* *Cancer of the Breast,* Statistical and Epidemiological Data, H. Seidman, MBA, American Cancer Society, Professional Education Publication.

The real solution to the problem, then, must lie in breast cancer prevention through vaccination, or in the *cure* of breast cancer through discovery of an effective anticancer drug or medication. Until such a time is reached, we must proceed as best we can with methods at hand, and we must be certain to follow a course leading to the greatest number of survivals. We must avoid preachments of faddists whose experience is meager, whose reasoning is fallacious, and whose statistics are based on inadequate samples.

The cause of breast cancer, as with so many other malignancies elsewhere in the body, is not known. We have mentioned several times that the high incidence of this disease in the breast is not unexpected. The breast is an organ in turmoil that must overcome the stresses and repeated fluctuations brought on by puberty, monthly menstrual periods, pregnancy, nursing, menopause, and the effects of taking hormones.

Pathologists now believe that the majority of breast cancers start out as cancers. However, they also believe that certain benign breast tumors have the potential to undergo malignant changes. These are known as *precancerous* lesions, the most prominent of which are considered to be cystic disease, cystosarcoma phyllodes, intraductal papillomas, intraductal hyperplasias, intraductal papillomatosis, and lobular neoplasia. But, as we have seen, it is impossible to tell before removing a benign lesion whether or not it is precancerous, and that therefore most physicians recommend that these lumps be excised as a precautionary measure. Also that intensive statistical surveys indicate that breast cancer is *not* inherited but that a definite tendency toward the development of this disease runs in some families.

It seems from these studies that a woman who is a member of a family with a grandmother, mother, or sister with breast cancer has *twice* the chance of getting the condition herself. (On the other hand, there is no predilection toward breast cancer in a woman who comes from a family with a high incidence of cancer in other organs of the body.) Statistically, the woman from a "breast cancer family" has about a one-in-seven chance of contracting the disease at some time in her life. Therefore, she should be especially conscientious about examining her breasts every month and seeing her doctor at regular intervals.

Breast cancer is extremely rare in women under 25 years of age. The greatest number of cases are seen between the ages of 40 and 55 years, after which there is a steady, slow decline in incidence for the remaining years of life. Haagensen's * statistics covering 6,000 cases over a 50-year period show the following ages of incidence:

Years of Age	Percent of Total Number of Cases
10 to 14	0
15 to 19	0
20 to 24	0.2
25 to 29	1.0
30 to 34	3.1
35 to 39	7.7
40 to 44	12.9
45 to 49	14.9
50 to 54	14.4
55 to 59	12.6
60 to 64	10.7
65 to 69	9.8
70 to 74	6.3
75 to 79	3.8
80 to 84	1.7
85 to 90	0.7
90 +	0.1

There has been considerable discussion of the possible benefits of nursing as a preventive of breast cancer. Statistics have come from various parts of the world that seem to indicate that there is a lower incidence of breast cancer in areas where women habitually breast-feed their offspring. In Israel, where the population is derived mainly from Europe and Asia, there is a striking difference between the incidence of cancer of the breast in the two groups. The incidence of breast cancer among the Jews of

* C. D. Haagensen, professor emeritus of breast surgery at Columbia–Presbyterian Medical Center in *Diseases of the Breast* (W. B. Saunders Co., Philadelphia, Pennsylvania).

European origin, where it is not customary to nurse newborn infants, is much greater than among the Jews of Asian origin, where breast-feeding is almost universal. Similar studies have revealed similar statistics in India, China, and Japan. How much added protection is afforded the woman who nurses her offspring cannot really be calculated, but it is known that the breast was designed to nurse, and an organ that fails to fulfill its function is more likely to become involved in a disease process. It is difficult to know whether the added protection against breast cancer outweighs the handicaps often caused by breast-feeding. A huge proportion of young women today must work for a living or must care for other children at home; and nursing can place a truly great burden on them. But women who come from families with a high incidence of breast cancer might do well to nurse their children.

Too much emphasis cannot be placed on the need for earlier diagnosis of breast cancer, but one of the great deterrents is the absence of pain as a symptom in this disease. It is a meaningful, dominant symptom in only 1 of 20 cases. By far the outstanding sign is a lump in the breast. In 95 percent of the cases, the lump is discovered by the woman herself. With intensified health education it is hoped that more women will practice self-examination, thus resulting in more lumps being found at an earlier stage of growth. Of course, the family physician is a key factor in early detection but he, too, must be educated to make breast examination a routine part of every examination he carries out on an adult female. Unfortunately, many doctors neglect to do this. And it is quite disquieting to record that a spouse is seldom the discoverer of a lump in his wife's breast. Other symptoms that occasionally give a clue to the presence of breast malignancy are discharge from the nipple, occurring in about 3 percent of women with this disease, retraction of the nipple, an ulceration of the nipple, enlargement of the breast, and changes in the appearance of the skin of the breast so that it resembles the skin of an orange.

A diagnosis of cancer can often be made merely by the manual examination of the breast, without the help of more sophisticated aids such as mammography, xeroradiography, or thermography. Quite naturally, a higher rate of accurate diagnosis is obtained when the breast is examined by an expert than when it is examined by a family doctor who sees relatively few patients with breast disease. Since every physician is anxious to be as accurate as possible, manual examination is seldom relied on as the sole method of diagnosis. If a suspicion of breast cancer exists, mammography, xeroradiography, thermography, needle biopsy, cytology, incisional biopsy, or excisional biopsy may be prescribed.

As for the patient, she is always interested to know how long an interval can safely elapse between the discovery of a lump and its definitive treatment. Naturally, the sooner the condition is taken care of, the better. However, it is not always possible to obtain a hospital bed, nor time in the operating-room schedule, as soon as one might wish. In many urban areas, hospital beds and a surgeon's available time are so completely occupied that patients must wait two to three weeks before they can be accommodated. In the life history of a breast cancer, two to three weeks is a brief time and studies have shown that a wait of this length does not alter the outcome of the disease. On the other hand, unnecessary waiting periods exceeding one month can only be conducive to further growth of the tumor and to its possible spread beyond the breast to the lymph nodes in the armpit. Moreover, the longer the preoperative waiting period, the greater the strain on the patient and her family.

As soon as it is decided to proceed surgically, discussions concerning the nature of the specific operation to be performed usually take place between the surgeon, the patient, and members of her family. Within recent years surgeons have come to realize that the patient and her family should play a greater role in decision making. Certainly, all the facts, theories, and possibilities should be brought out into the open and discussed fully. *It is the obligation of the surgeon to tell his patient and her family the current thinking of the great majority of surgeons concerning how to secure the greatest numbers of survivals and cures. They should be told the conclusions reached by organizations such as the American Cancer Society, by the great cancer institutions such as Memorial Hospital in New York and Roswell Park in Buffalo, and by the overwhelming majority of specialists in the field of breast surgery whose statistics are based upon thousands, not dozens, of cases.*

The personal theories and hypothecations of a small group of those performing breast surgery, whose statistics are based on small samples, should not determine the type of treatment the average woman undergoes for her breast cancer. To tell a patient with breast cancer that her chances for survival are just as good even if part of the cancer (which could be easily excised) is left behind, borders on the ridiculous. To tell her this when the data are based on a few hundred cases (rather than the tens of thousands of cases that have been analyzed by the American Cancer Society and university hospitals throughout the country), is the height of unscientific thinking. Of course, women want to hear that their breast can be saved. And, if they are informed that their chances for cure are just as great with mere removal of the lump, or removing only part of the breast, naturally, they will be inclined to accept these methods of treatment.

In more than forty years of breast surgery, I have encountered less than a handful of patients who, on being told of a possible cancer, wanted to have each and every contemplated procedure explained in detail before submitting to surgery. Invariably, they want to know whether or not it will be necessary to remove the breast. They are terribly concerned about this possibility, but care little whether the muscles of the chest wall or the lymph nodes in the armpit will or will not be excised. To expect a patient, no matter how highly educated and intelligent she may be, to understand the comparative worths of radical mastectomy vs. modified radical mastectomy vs. simple mastectomy vs. partial mastectomy vs. lumpectomy—or to evaluate her chances for survival or cure with one or the other operation— is sheer nonsense. And to expect her to make a meaningful evaluation at a time when she is so emotionally upset by the news that she has breast cancer is asking the impossible! If *her* decision was binding, and if it differed from her surgeon's recommendation, it might very well cost her her life.

"Radical" Mastectomy

The term *radical* has peculiar connotations, mainly because of its usage in the political sense. Radical also stands for something drastic, wild, uncontrolled. Thus, if there is an operation that is not *radical* that can accomplish equally good results, most people are for it. However, in the medical sense, the word radical stands for thorough or complete. As examples, there are operations known as "Radical Neck Dissection," "Radical Groin Dissection," "Radical Hysterectomy," "Radical Mastoidectomy," and so on. In each instance, the word *radical* stands for *thorough* or *complete,* as opposed to *simple* or *incomplete.*

Thorough (radical) mastectomy, carried out by the great majority

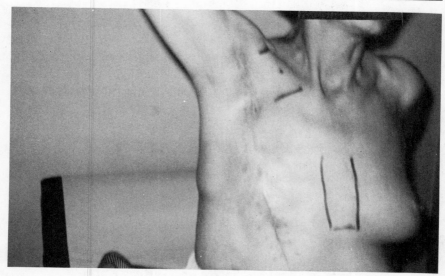

Recent thorough (radical) mastectomy showing markings for administration of postoperative cobalt therapy.

of American surgeons as the most effective treatment for resectable breast cancer, includes removal of the breast with the underlying pectoral muscles of the chest wall and the lymph nodes along the blood vessels below the collarbone, in the armpit (axilla), and along the lateral chest wall. It is carried out through a breast-encircling incision either in a vertical or horizontal plane. The skin in all directions surrounding the incision is undermined so as to permit it to come together after the breast has been removed. If the edges of the incision cannot be brought together at the completion of the operation, a thin skin graft is taken from the patient's thigh and is transferred to the bare area on the chest wall.

Thorough mastectomy may require anywhere from two to six or more hours to perform, depending on specific technical problems that are encountered during the dissection and the rate of speed at which the particular surgeon works. The thoroughness of the procedure does not necessarily depend on the pace, fast or slow, at which the surgeon works, nor is the patient often sicker after a slow operation than after a rapid one. Operative recovery following thorough mastectomy is the general rule.

Extended Thorough (Radical) Mastectomy

This operation includes the removal of all the tissues excised during the course of the standard thorough mastectomy plus the lymph nodes of the internal mammary chain. These nodes, usually four to six in number, are located beneath the edge of the breastbone at the level of the second, third, fourth, and fifth ribs. The procedure, also known as the Urban operation,* is limited to those patients who have a cancer on that portion of the breast nearest to the midline. The operation has not been routinely adopted because it is felt that if cancer has spread to these nodes, the disease is too far advanced to lend itself to surgical eradication. Despite this contention, in Dr. Urban's hands the end results appear to offer greater survival rates than if the standard thorough mastectomy is performed.

Modified Thorough (Radical) Mastectomy

This operation involves the removal of the entire breast through the same incisions used for the standard thorough mastectomy, but it does not remove the pectoral muscles of the anterior chest wall. Surgeons who advocate this procedure claim to be able to remove as many of the lymph nodes as those who perform the standard operation. They also claim that the visible chest wall disfigurement is lessened by the operation, that the patient has greater use of her arm, and that end results are just as good with this as with the unmodified procedure.

It has been my experience that even when the lymph nodes are removed, cancer may lurk in the tissue (fascia) surrounding the pectoral muscles or in difficult-to-find small lymph nodes lying between the two pectoral muscles.

In 1966, I operated on a 51-year-old woman with a large breast cancer and involvement of every one of the twenty-one lymph nodes found in the axilla. The pathologist also reported five involved lymph nodes in the pectoral fascia. A standard thorough mastectomy was performed

---

* Named for Dr. J. A. Urban, attending breast surgeon, Memorial Sloan-Kettering Hospital, New York.

and, to date, the patient is well and clinically free of cancer. If the pectoral muscles had been left behind in this case, in all probability, the involved lymph nodes and involved surrounding connective tissues would have remained behind. Naturally this patient would not be free of cancer today.

Most surgeons in this country agree that it is technically more difficult to perform a thorough operation when leaving behind the pectoral muscles. They also believe that the advantage in retaining the muscles is more cosmetic than functional, because most women have practically full use of their arms after removal of the pectorals. Whatever advantage there is to the modified operation is outweighed by the added risk of leaving behind cancerous nodes and tissues.

Simple Mastectomy

In simple mastectomy the entire breast is removed down to, but not including, the pectoral muscles. The lymph nodes beneath the collarbone, in the armpit, and alongside the breast are left intact. The majority of surgeons in this country reserve simple mastectomy to poor surgical risk patients, to those who are far advanced in age (in their eighth decade), and to those whose cancer has spread beyond the reach of the scalpel. Surgery in this latter group is usually carried out only for the purpose of excising a cancer that has ulcerated, or to reduce the amount of cancer tissue in the body so that chemotherapy will be more effective. (It has been found that the smaller the size of the tumor or the less the amount of tumor tissue that has spread to other parts of the body, the more effective is chemotherapy.)

A considerable number of surgeons in Europe, and a small group in the United States, believe that results with simple mastectomy, either with or without postoperative X-ray or cobalt therapy, are just as good as those following thorough (radical) mastectomy. They base their claims on five-year survival rates which the following chart contradicts (even without surgery of any kind the survival rate of the average breast cancer patient from the time she is first seen approaches four years).

An interesting study of survival after thorough (radical) mastectomy versus that after modified thorough (radical) mastectomy versus that after simple mastectomy was carried out at the Buffalo General Hospital in

Buffalo, New York.* It showed that survival after any one of the three operations was similar for the first two years, but thereafter through 20 years, *the patients with the least surgical intervention did the worst and those with "radical" operations did the best.*

Years of Survival	Percent Survival with Thorough (Radical) Mastectomy	Percent Survival with Modified Thorough (Radical) Mastectomy	Percent Survival with Simple Mastectomy
5 years	66	53	46
10 years	52	41	31
15 years	41	35	24

The above statistics include those patients with, as well as those without, spread of the cancer to neighboring lymph nodes. The three groups are quite similar, state the authors, insofar as tumor size and lymph node involvement is concerned.

In the hands of Haagensen, 10-year survival rates after thorough (radical) mastectomy were 62 percent, whereas the 10-year survival rate following simple mastectomy, as presented in a report entitled, "Cooperative International Comparison of the Treatment of Early Carcinoma," was only 37 percent.

Partial Mastectomy

Partial mastectomy involves wide local removal of the quadrant of the breast in which the cancer is located. A diamond-shaped segment of overlying fat tissue and skin is removed along with the cancer-bearing portion of the breast. In some cases, underlying tissues covering the pectoral muscles are included in the dissection. After excision of these tissues, an attempt is made to restore the appearance of the breast. Those few surgeons who advocate this operation for breast cancer limit its use to cancers in the outer portion of the breast. *Those who perform this type*

* G. H. Leah, J. Berg, E. H. Wesp, G. F. Robbins, writing in *Surgery, Gynecology & Obstetrics,* November 1969.

of surgery in an attempt to cure cancer are playing Russian roulette with their patients' lives. They ignore the fact that in 6 out of 10 cancers, the cancer exists in several other places within the breast, even though a lump cannot be felt. Thus, in 60 percent of cases they needlessly leave cancer behind to grow and to kill.

Lumpectomy

Lumpectomy is a lay term coined by surgeons who perform partial mastectomy. The operation involves wide local excision of the cancer, followed by irradiation. Lumpectomy removes less tissue than partial mastectomy. This is not Russian roulette. All but one chamber is filled with live bullets!

Surgeons who advise partial mastectomy or lumpectomy as a definitive treatment for breast cancer base their claims upon meager samples—in some instances no more than 10 percent of those made available for statistical review by the American Cancer Society and some of the large institutions that specialize in the treatment of cancer. Moreover, since the average breast cancer patient will survive for approximately 4 years after she is first seen, no matter which form of surgical treatment is rendered, these doctors might just as well advocate needle biopsy as a definitive form of treatment of this disease. Their patients survive not because of the lumpectomy or partial mastectomy, but because of the postoperative irradiation, chemotherapy, and hormone therapy they receive.

As for the contention that cancer, acting as a foreign body, stimulates the formation of antibodies, evidence is growing that there may be some truth to this theory. An extension of this theory is that perhaps cancerous lymph nodes in the armpit may inhibit growth of cancer cells that have gotten into the bloodstream and have traveled to distant parts of the body. There may be some truth to this contention, too. However, in our present state of immunological knowledge on this subject, there is far greater risk in leaving behind cancer that can be removed than there is gain from supposed immune reactions of an undetermined nature.

* * *

It is difficult to follow the process of reasoning among those who advocate simple rather than thorough (radical) mastectomy. Surely, the immediate mortality rate is the same for both operations. As far as the

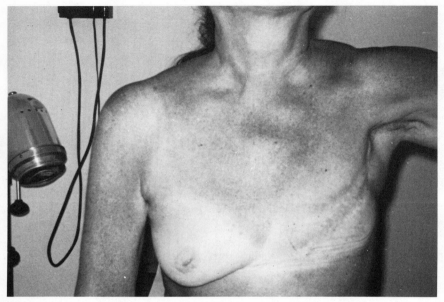

Incisions for thorough (radical) mastectomy can be so placed that they will not be seen when the woman wears an evening dress or bathing suit.

scars are concerned, thorough mastectomy does create somewhat more disfigurement than simple mastectomy, but the potential advantages from removing *all* rather than part of the cancer more than compensate for the added scars. It must be admitted that the patient who has undergone thorough mastectomy will have more pain in the chest area, the shoulder, the arm, and in the back than one who has had simple mastectomy. This is a price one must pay for thorough mastectomy, but if a woman looks at the Buffalo General Hospital statistics in the preceding table, she will see that she is well repaid in longevity for the added discomfort.

Of course simple mastectomy is an adequate operation for women who have no spread of the cancer to the neighboring lymph nodes. However, it is impossible to know without removing them whether they are or are not cancerous. Inspection and manual palpation of the nodes is totally inadequate. There are anywhere from fifteen to fifty lymph nodes draining the areas immediately adjacent to the breast, and few of them come into view when performing simple mastectomy. Even if they did, inspection would not tell the story, as some of the smallest nodes may be involved in cancer.

One of the main reasons to prefer simple over thorough mastectomy is postoperative edema (swelling) of the arm. This is a most troublesome sequel of axillary (armpit) dissection. It is present to a lesser or greater degree in about one out of four patients who have undergone thorough mastectomy. However, edema, which increases the circumference of the upper arm by more than two inches or the forearm by more than an inch, occurs in only about 10 percent of the cases. This condition will be discussed further in another chapter.

To test the wisdom of lumpectomy and partial mastectomy, the Breast Surgical Service at the Memorial Sloan-Kettering Hospital carried out a study upon 508 breast cancer patients admitted to the hospital and subjected to surgery during a two-year period.* They removed the cancers with a wide local excision, making their line of excision at least twice the size of the tumor mass (and almost the size of what would have been removed during lumpectomy or some partial mastectomies). These specimens were then submitted to the laboratory for microscopic diagnosis. When the report was received that cancer was present, the Memorial Hospital surgeons proceeded with the removal of the entire breast. *After completion of the mastectomy, the excised breast was also sent to the laboratory, and in 59 percent of the patients, residual cancer was found, near or distant to the site where the local excision had been carried out. In other words, if lumpectomy or partial mastectomy had been the total operation, cancer would have been left behind needlessly in 6 out of every 10 of their patients.*

As stated earlier, the above finding is not unexpected. Cancer of the breast is frequently multicentric. This means that it arises from several different areas within the same breast. Therefore, the excision of anything less than the whole breast is inadequate treatment.

To obtain a broader picture of current thought on the type of surgery that should be performed for cancer of the breast, I questioned all the chairmen of the surgical departments in our American medical schools. Specifically, they were asked to comment on the idea that lesser operations

---

* J. P. Shah, P. P. Rosen, G. F. Robbins, writing in *Surgery, Gynecology & Obstetrics*, May 1973. (Their sample was 10 times larger than that used by the "lumpectomy" surgeons.)

such as modified thorough (radical) mastectomy, simple mastectomy, partial mastectomy, and lumpectomy could bring about just as good survival rates as the standard thorough (radical) mastectomy. Forty professors of surgery replied, and 33 of them, or 82.5 percent, thought that thorough (radical) mastectomy offered the best chances for cure in breast cancer; 7 thought that a modified thorough (radical) mastectomy could accomplish the same results. None advocated partial mastectomy or lumpectomy as the operation of choice for patients with cancer of the breast.

Postoperative Irradiation

After any operation for breast cancer, it is necessary to decide whether postoperative irradiation should be given. Postoperative irradiation is definitely beneficial in that it can kill cancer cells that may have been inadvertently left behind when performing a mastectomy. It is therefore frequently recommended in cases of breast cancer associated with lymph node involvement as well as in cases where less than maximum operations have been performed.

Today, such therapy consists of cobalt or high voltage X-ray radiation. Most surgeons advocate postoperative irradiation for patients who have, at operation, shown cancerous involvement of the lymph nodes in the armpit, in the region of the collarbone or base of the neck, in the area lateral to the breast, or in the nodes beneath the breastbone. They do not advocate postoperative X-ray or cobalt therapy if the lymph nodes are found to be free of cancer. Postoperative irradiation is given because some cancer cells may be left behind despite the most thorough surgical dissection. The irradiation will in many instances destroy these cells.

Surgeons who routinely perform simple mastectomy or lesser operations as definitive treatment for breast cancer are more likely to rely on postoperative irradiation to contain the growth of tumor cells that might be growing in the nodes they have left behind. The need to irradiate is another argument in favor of thorough mastectomy over simple mastectomy. When the thorough procedure has been followed, the surgeon knows definitely whether or not the lymph nodes are cancerous, and he therefore knows whether or not irradiation will be necessary. In lesser operations, the surgeon can only guess about lymph node involvement.

The patient is spared a great deal of expense and discomfort if she can avoid postoperative irradiation. In the average case, she must go to the radiologist's office every weekday for approximately six weeks. Moreover, there are distressing side effects such as nausea, loss of appetite, irritation of the skin, and a general feeling of malaise in many women who are undergoing X-ray or cobalt therapy. And, finally, some patients who have had intensive radiation therapy to the chest area develop fibrosis of the lungs, with an annoying, uncontrollable, dry, hacking cough.

Postoperative Hormone Therapy

Hormone therapy—usually male sex hormone (androgen) for younger women and female sex hormone (stilbestrol) for older women—is reserved for those who have a local or distant recurrence of their cancer. The lifespan can often be extended for several months or years by the judicious treatment with the appropriate hormone, even when the malignancy has invaded distant organs. Frequently, the hormones are given in conjunction with anticancer chemicals.

Ablative Surgery

Ablative (to remove by cutting out) surgery is recommended for some patients whose breast cancer has metastasized, or spread, to distant parts of the body or has recurred locally. If the woman is of premenopausal age, removal of the ovaries (oophorectomy) is recommended. This procedure causes a remission in the growth of the tumor in some 30 to 40 percent of cases. The remission may last from several months to two to three years. If the metastases grow again, adrenalectomy (removal of the adrenal glands) or hypophysectomy (removal of the pituitary gland in the base of the brain) may be indicated. Remissions following these procedures occur in approximately half the cases *if* they had responded favorably to removal of the ovaries. A lack of response to removal of the ovaries often indicates that there will be an equally unfavorable response after adrenalectomy or hypophysectomy.

Adrenalectomy and hypophysectomy are sometimes successful in obtaining remissions of several months to several years duration in those patients who are past the menopause and therefore were not subjected to removal of their ovaries.

Unfortunately, cure of breast cancer does not result from these operations and many physicians doubt their advisability. They feel that the temporary prolongation of life wrought by these operative procedures is not worth the additional suffering and postoperative complications that so frequently accompany their use. Certainly, ablative surgery should never be undertaken unless it is fully discussed with the patient and she gives her full, informed consent.

Postoperative Chemotherapy

Progress in the field of anticancer drugs has been marvelously rapid and successful within the past few years. Advances have been so great that an ever-increasing number of physicians now advocate the routine postoperative use of chemotherapy for those patients whose cancer has involved the lymph nodes adjacent to the breast. Indeed, many specialists in this field are of the opinion that a course of postoperative chemotherapy should replace the use of X-ray or cobalt therapy as a means of killing cancer cells that may remain behind after surgery. They point to the fact that the anticancer chemicals go to every part of the body where cancer cells may have spread, whereas postoperative X rays or cobalt merely attack those cells in the localized region of the chest and armpit.

Recent studies tend to show a markedly decreased incidence of recurrence of cancer among those women who have undergone a thorough course of chemotherapy with drugs known as L-PAM and Adriamycin. It is not possible, at the time of this writing, to give definitive statistics on the ultimate outcome of this method of treatment, as a ten-year period has not yet elapsed since its inauguration. Moreover, it has not yet been determined that chemotherapy alone is a better approach than chemotherapy *plus* X-ray or cobalt irradiation, or chemotherapy *plus* hormone or ablative therapy, or a combination of all three methods of combating cancer that has spread beyond the local confines of the breast.

Chemotherapy for breast cancer must be carried out only by experts in the field, who must work in close association with the surgeon, radiologist, and endocrinologist. And since anticancer chemicals have a tendency to inhibit the production of the white blood cells that combat infection, it is essential that chemotherapists work in close consultation with the hematologist. By this team approach, the maximum number of postoperative patients can be spared the recurrence of cancer, and a maximum amount of prolongation of life can be obtained for those who suffer from breast cancer that has already spread to other organs of the body.

Recurrence of Breast Cancer

A certain percentage of patients will develop a local or distant recurrence of breast cancer within the years following their surgery. Most recurrences take place within the first seven years after surgery, although a small number of patients may experience recurrence ten, twenty, or more years later. It is surmised that the metastatic cancer cells lie dormant until some unknown stimulant causes them to awaken and grow.

A woman who has had one breast cancer is approximately twice as prone to develop a cancer in the opposite breast. Since all women have approximately a one-in-fourteen chance of getting this disease, the patient who has survived cancer in one breast has a one-in-seven chance of getting it on the other side. With this knowledge in mind, she should certainly take every precaution to spot a tumor as early as possible. A visit to her surgeon every four months, monthly self-examination, mammography twice a year, possibly thermography twice a year, are all advisable for the post-mastectomy patient.

Recently, some surgeons have been taking random biopsies of the remaining breast in the mirror-image area of the original cancer in the opposite breast. Thus, if a woman had a cancer in the upper outer quadrant of the right breast, a biopsy is taken of tissue in the upper outer quadrant of the left breast. This procedure is based on the assumption that the cancer might be caused by some developmental deviation occurring during embryonic life. As a consequence, a likelihood exists that the defect would be bilateral. Although a sufficient number of cases has not been reported, it is interesting to learn that cancers are from time to time uncovered in this manner long before they appear clinically as a lump in the breast.

Also, local recurrences beneath the skin in the area of mastectomy are sometimes encountered. These recurrences signify in more than half the cases that the malignant process has also spread to distant organs. Despite this statistic, it is worthwhile to widely excise local recurrences as they may *not* represent anything more than a few cells left behind in the skin or subcutaneous tissues following the original surgery. In general, the longer the lapse of time between mastectomy and the appearance of a local recurrence, the better the prognosis.

Prognosis in Breast Cancer

A great number of factors govern the survival and cure rates in breast cancer. Some of the most important of these factors are:

1. Interval between time of tumor appearance and surgery. There is no doubt that the earlier a tumor is removed, the better are the chances for cure. All studies indicate that the longer the interval between discovery of a lump and its ultimate removal, the lower will be the 5- and 10-year survival rates.

2. The size of the tumor when operated on. The smaller the tumor when removed, the more favorable are the 5- and 10-year survival rates.

3. Cancers located in the outer one-third of the breast have a better prognosis than those nearer to the center or toward the inner side of the breast.

4. Tumors located in, or originating from, the ducts of the breast that have not spread out into distant parts of the breast have a better prognosis than those that have disseminated throughout the breast.

5. Tumors that are unicentric, originating from one spot, usually have a better prognosis than cancers that are multicentric, originating simultaneously in several areas within the breast.

6. Tumors that have not involved surrounding lymph nodes have a much better prognosis than tumors that have already invaded surrounding nodes. The fewer the involved lymph nodes, the better the prognosis, provided thorough (radical) mastectomy has been performed.

7. Pathological classification of breast cancer has some bearing on prognosis, but it is less important than clinical classification. A tumor that, upon microscopic examination, appears to be rapidly growing and exceptionally malignant carries with it a poorer prognosis than a slow-growing tumor

or a *carcinoma in situ,* the latter being a cancer that is non-invasive and confined.

8(a). Cytological examination of individual breast cancer cells has recently given strong clues as to prognosis. This examination requires the study of the cells to note the absence or presence of so-called *Barr bodies* within the cytoplasm. Barr bodies are seen as small dots in the outer rim of the cancer cells. If, after counting 500 cells, there are less than 30 percent of cells showing Barr bodies, the prognosis is poor. If there are 30 to 50 percent of cells showing the Barr bodies, the prognosis is fair. If more than 50 percent of cells show the characteristic Barr bodies, the prognosis is good. The examination requires over 2 hours to perform, and must be carried out on a freshly removed specimen by an expert cytologist.

(b). It has been known for some time that certain breast cancers are *estrogen-dependent,* whereas others are not. Recently, a chemical test has been evolved whereby the "estrogen binding capacity" of a breast tumor can be ascertained. If the estrogen binding capacity is low, the prognosis is good; if the estrogen binding capacity is high, the prognosis is poor. This test is in the research stage and cannot yet be used as a reliable guide to prognosis.

*　*　*

Before terminating this discussion, it should be emphasized that early detection of existing cancer is not the entire answer to the breast problem. *We must seek out, identify, and zone-in on the 90,000 women who do not now have breast cancer but who will develop one next year, or during the years after next year.* We want to know NOW, when the breasts are cancer-free but cancer-prone, who these women are. We want to forewarn them, study them, and perhaps treat them *before* they develop a breast cancer.

The task of locating and identifying this group of cancer-prone patients is a great one, but much can be done toward that end within the framework of our present knowledge. A great many of the 4,590,000 women now alive in the United States who will one day develop breast cancer fall into one or more of the following categories:

1. They are women with cystic disease of the breasts who have undergone more than one operation for the condition.
2. They are women with widespread ductal hyperplasia, as proven by surgical biopsy.
3. They are women who have undergone surgery for an intraductal papilloma.
4. They are women who have undergone surgery for intraductal papillomatosis.
5. They are women who have undergone surgery for lobular neoplasia.
6. They are women who have cystic disease, intraductal hyperplasia, an intraductal papilloma, intraductal papillomatosis, or lobular neoplasia but have not been treated for their condition.
7. They have a history of breast cancer in a mother, sister, or grandmother.

These women must, of course, be urged to practice self-examination each month, to undergo breast examination by a surgeon every four months, and to have mammography and thermography twice a year. But this is not enough! Should any woman who comes from a breast cancer family show any signs of new or persistent breast pathology as described above, one or more of the following procedures should be given serious consideration:

1. Cobalt radiation or surgical removal of the ovaries, if the woman is finished with childbearing but is still having menstrual periods. (It is well documented that approximately half of all breast cancers are hormone-dependent. Thus, removal of the hormones through radiation or removal of the ovaries could remove some of the stimulus to breast cancer development.)
2. The performance of a subcutaneous mastectomy for those women in this group who come from a breast cancer family and who have had more than one operation for the breast diseases listed above. (Breast contours would be restored by the insertion of silastic bags.)
3. Although a course of chemotherapy has not yet been advocated as a means of destroying cells that are precancerous, this eventuality might not be too far distant. As a first step,

the effect of some of the newer chemicals upon areas of breast tissue involved in lobular neoplasia might be ascertained.

Questions and Answers

Does breast-feeding help to prevent the ultimate development of breast cancer?

It is thought that the incidence of breast cancer is lower among women who nurse their children but it has not been clearly calculated just how much protection is afforded by breast-feeding. Nursing one infant certainly has less influence on the breast than nursing five or six offspring.

Will the giving of female sex hormones increase the chances of developing breast cancer?

No, although it may stimulate cystic disease or nipple discharge. Despite specific knowledge on this subject, women from breast cancer families had best avoid the use of female sex hormones.

Will the taking of birth control pills over a long period of time lead toward the development of breast cancer?

No, although it may stimulate cystic disease or nipple discharge. Here, too, women from breast cancer families are better advised not to use birth control pills.

Does cancer ever take place during pregnancy?
Yes, but it is rare.

Should the pregnancy be interrupted if a breast cancer is found?

It depends on the stage of fetal development when the breast cancer is found. If it is found in early pregnancy, the pregnancy should be interrupted. If it is discovered when the fetus is viable, the pregnancy should not be interrupted. The important thing is to remove the cancerous breast as promptly as possible.

What is the expectation of complete cure for the type of breast cancer seen during pregnancy?

This type of cancer constitutes the most virulent form of the disease. However, better results with longer survival rates are now being obtained with prompt mastectomy.

Can a surgeon tell that a breast cancer is too far advanced for surgery to be helpful?

Yes, if there are involved lymph nodes above the collarbone or in the chest cavity. Also, X rays may show spread of the cancer into the bones or other organs in far advanced cases.

Are special nurses necessary following major breast surgery?

They are not necessary, but the patient will derive great comfort from them if she can afford their cost.

Can a surgeon tell whether there has been a spread of the cancer into the lymph nodes under the armpit before he operates?

He can tell whether or not they are enlarged, and if they are, he may surmise that they are involved in cancer. However, he is frequently wrong! The nodes may be enlarged due to inflammation, not cancer.

Can a surgeon tell at the operating table whether the glands under the armpit are involved in cancer?

Yes, usually. However, even small, innocent-appearing nodes may harbor cancer cells. A final determination of node involvement must await the pathologist's examination. This may take several days.

How long is one in the hospital following thorough (radical) mastectomy?

From seven to twelve days.

How long is one in the hospital following simple mastectomy?

From seven to nine days.

What are the chances for a complete cure for breast cancer?

Slightly more than four out of five women with cancer of the breast can be saved if it is discovered before the tumor has spread beyond the breast. The percentage would be even higher were it not for the fact that so few patients seek advice early in the course of their disease. (The mortality for men with cancer of the breast is somewhat greater than for women.) If the cancer has, at the time of surgery, spread to the glands in the armpit, survival rates are reduced by approximately 50 percent.

Is there a possibility of a "cure" even though the cancer has spread to the nodes in the armpit?

Yes, but the "cure" rate is reduced to about half of that found in patients without lymph node involvement.

Are the number of lymph nodes that are involved a factor in predicting survival?

Yes, the general rule is that the more glands in the armpit that are involved in cancer, the fewer chances there are for total recovery. However, if only one or two glands of the thirty or forty that are present are involved, the chances for cure are still great.

Is the prognosis better if the lymph nodes high in the axilla (armpit) are uninvolved?

Yes.

How long does it take the wound to heal after a thorough (radical) mastectomy?

Approximately 2 to 3 weeks.

How long does it take to convalesce from thorough (radical) mastectomy?

Usually 4 to 6 weeks. The arm on the involved side may require special physical therapy, and in certain instances, this must continue for several months postoperatively. It must be understood that complete recovery includes the acceptance of a certain amount of pain and discomfort in the operative area.

Is it natural for the chest wall to feel tight and painful following thorough (radical) mastectomy?

Yes.

For how long does pain remain following thorough (radical) mastectomy?

It may last several weeks, months, or even years, depending on the individual's sensitivity to pain.

Is numbness and tingling in the chest wall, shoulder, back, and arm a natural phenomenon after breast removal?

Yes, in many cases.

Do numbness and tingling tend to disappear after a period of time?
Yes, but it may require several months.

Does the tightness and constriction found in the chest tend to disappear?
Yes, but it may require several months.

Should a woman regain full use of her arm following thorough (radical) mastectomy?
Yes.

Can a woman comb her hair as easily as she used to following breast removal?
At first it may be difficult, but eventually she will be able to do so.

What is postoperative edema (swelling) of the arm?
The type that occurs immediately following thorough (radical) mastectomy.

What is secondary edema of the arm?
It is a swelling that comes on after the wound has healed. It tends to persist indefinitely.

What causes swelling of the arm after thorough (radical) mastectomy?
Interruption of the lymphatic channels and removal of the glands (nodes) that drain the lymph from the arm. It is thought that wound infection, a complication in some cases, contributes toward the edema.

Can one predict beforehand who will develop a swollen arm after mastectomy and who will not develop this complication?
No.

Can one prevent the swelling of the arm that sometimes takes place after thorough (radical) mastectomy?
No, except that those who perform a careful axillary dissection and those who are most scrupulous in avoiding operative wound infection seem to have the lowest incidence of postoperative edema.

What is the treatment for swelling of the arm following thorough (radical) mastectomy?
See chapter 29.

Will the swelling of the arm tend to disappear after a time?
Only to a minor extent.

Does swelling of the arm ever take place after simple mastectomy?
No.

Should a woman be particularly careful to avoid infection in an arm on the side of a thorough (radical) mastectomy?
Yes, because an infection may lead to the development of edema.

How soon after mastectomy can a woman be fitted for a brassiere?
Within two to three weeks.

How soon after mastectomy can a woman resume marital relations?
As soon as the wound has healed. From a psychological point of view, the sooner this occurs, the better. Women who wait too long may develop unnecessary inhibitions.

How soon after a thorough (radical) mastectomy can a patient get out of bed?
Within 24 hours.

Can a woman permit herself to become pregnant after she has had a mastectomy for cancer of the breast?
In all probability, this is unwise. However, if she has been free of recurrence for 7 or more years, it may be all right for her to become pregnant.

Does cancer ever subside by itself?
No.

How long will a patient survive with untreated breast cancer?
There have been many studies in this regard but most of them tend to show that the average duration of life in these patients is approximately 3½ years from the time of the first knowledge that a cancer is present.

29 PHYSICAL RECOVERY FROM BREAST SURGERY

Most patients who have undergone breast surgery are spared many of the truly distressing postoperative measures to which other patients are subjected. They require no tubes in their stomachs, no catheters in their bladders, and no prolonged intubation of their windpipes. Intravenous infusions can be discontinued within twenty-four hours and the patient can resume a regular diet. Some mastectomy patients, however, may require intravenous infusions for a few days as their ability to take sufficient nourishment may be inhibited by the nausea and lack of appetite which frequently follow a prolonged anesthesia and operation.

Within four to six days, drains are removed in mastectomy patients and they are up and about, eating a full diet. *However, from the first day after surgery, the nurse and surgeon must insist that she raise the arm on the involved side despite the pain it may produce.* This must be carried out several times each day so that no adhesions, limiting motion of the arm, begin to form. A full range of motion is rarely possible at this early stage, but every postoperative mastectomy patient should be able to raise her upper arm above a 45° angle from the very start.

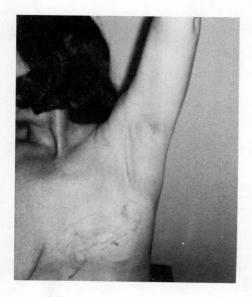

Extent of arm movement three years after thorough mastectomy.

All women who have had a breast removed are urged to start regular exercises to ensure the return of a full range of motion and to strengthen the muscles of their shoulder and arm. These exercises should be a continuation of the exercises begun in the hospital. They should be carried out at least 6 times daily; on arising in the morning, between breakfast and lunch, at lunchtime, between lunchtime and dinner, at dinnertime, and before retiring. Women should not go beyond the point of their endurance in performing the exercises nor should they do them so briefly as to miss any possible benefit from their performance. They will find that as time passes, they will be able to continue each set of exercises for a longer period of time before tiring.

Patients not infrequently become lax about doing their exercises during the period when they may be going for daily radiotherapy treatments or receiving chemotherapy. This is a mistake, and even though they are tired and may feel ill from the effects of the treatments, it is essential that they continue their exercises. Adhesions are most likely to form just during the period when irradiation is in progress. If exercises are neglected during these weeks, permanent limitation of motion may result.

The Reach to Recovery Program recommends the following exercises. In my experience, they have been most effective.

WALL CLIMBING AND MEASUREMENT

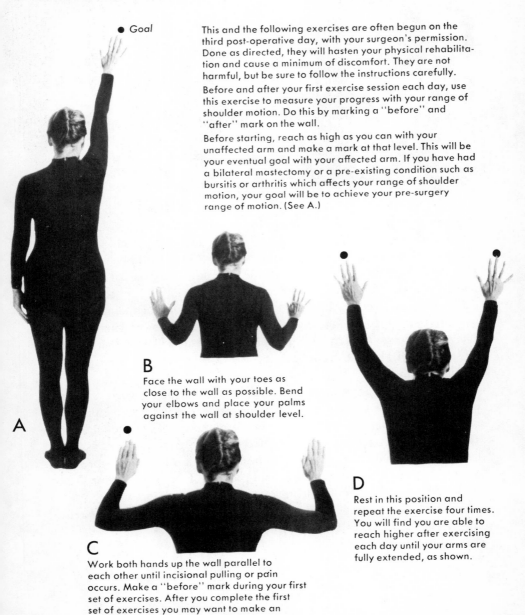

● *Goal*

This and the following exercises are often begun on the third post-operative day, with your surgeon's permission. Done as directed, they will hasten your physical rehabilitation and cause a minimum of discomfort. They are not harmful, but be sure to follow the instructions carefully.

Before and after your first exercise session each day, use this exercise to measure your progress with your range of shoulder motion. Do this by marking a "before" and "after" mark on the wall.

Before starting, reach as high as you can with your unaffected arm and make a mark at that level. This will be your eventual goal with your affected arm. If you have had a bilateral mastectomy or a pre-existing condition such as bursitis or arthritis which affects your range of shoulder motion, your goal will be to achieve your pre-surgery range of motion. (See A.)

A

B
Face the wall with your toes as close to the wall as possible. Bend your elbows and place your palms against the wall at shoulder level.

C
Work both hands up the wall parallel to each other until incisional pulling or pain occurs. Make a "before" mark during your first set of exercises. After you complete the first set of exercises you may want to make an "after" mark to measure your progress.

D
Rest in this position and repeat the exercise four times. You will find you are able to reach higher after exercising each day until your arms are fully extended, as shown.

EXERCISE **2**

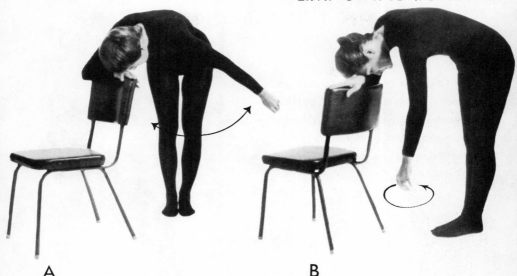

A

Place your un-
affected arm on the
back of a chair and rest your
forehead on that arm. Slowly
allow your affected arm (the
operated side) to hang loosely
until your elbow is straight and
the whole arm and hand are limp.

Swing your arm limply from left
to right within a comfortable
range making sure the motion
comes from your shoulder and
not your elbow. Swing until your
arm is relaxed.

B

Swing your arm in small circles,
again making sure the motion
comes from your shoulder. As
your arm relaxes, increase the
size of the circles staying within
your range of comfort. Reverse
the direction of the circles.

C

Swing your arm forward and
backward, from the shoulder.

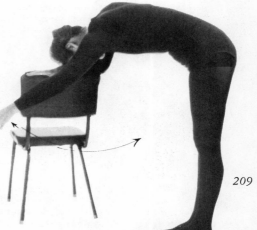

209

EXAGGERATED DEEP BREATHING

This exercise helps your posture and your
lungs, eases the feeling of tight skin or pressure
over your chest and relieves the pulling and
pain that may be caused by reaching in
the following exercises. Do this exercise
frequently.

Place the hand most comfortable
to use over the center of your chest.

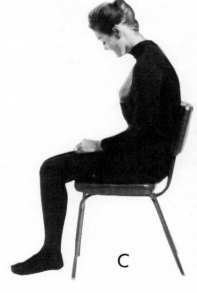

A

Take a slow, deep breath through
your nose and let your chest
expand fully.

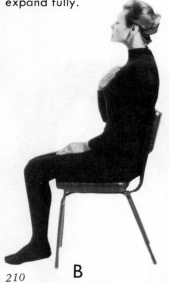

C

Exhale completely and let
your chest and shoulders
sag and relax.

B

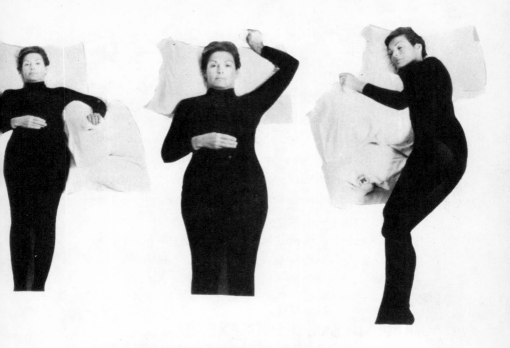

HAND SQUEEZING AND
POSITIONS FOR REST AND SLEEP

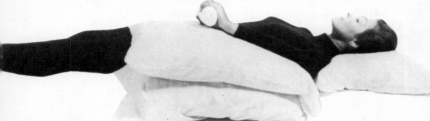

Immediately after surgery, you should begin squeezing a gauze roll or the rubber ball that you'll find in your Reach to Recovery kit. Your arm should be elevated as high as is comfortable on pillows to promote lymphatic drainage and reduce or prevent post-operative arm swelling.

Continue this elevation-squeezing combination as long as there is a tendency for your arm or hand to swell or there is a feeling of heaviness.

Later, when sitting on a couch, you should place your arm at shoulder level along the back of the couch and squeeze the ball in this position.

MIRROR EXERCISE

Good posture is vital to prevent a drooping shoulder or raised shoulder on the operated side. Stand before your mirror frequently to make certain your shoulders are even. Make a conscious effort to square your shoulders by rolling them back and keeping your arms down. This exercise will relax you and help minimize the hollow that may develop below your collar bone.

HAIR-BRUSHING EXERCISE

It is especially important for your morale to keep yourself looking pretty. Wear an attractive robe or housecoat, take time with your hair-do and makeup.

About four days after surgery, you may begin the hair-brushing exercise. Start by sitting beside a night table and resting your affected arm on a pile of books. Comb and brush your hair keeping your head erect.

One side is enough in the beginning. Gradually release your arm from its resting position and work the brush around your head until you have covered your entire scalp. Stop when you feel incisional pulling.

EXERCISE **4**

CLASP, REACH AND SPREAD

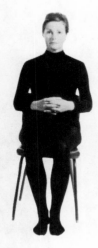

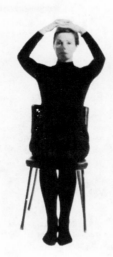

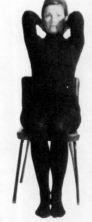

A

Sit up straight and clasp your hands together.

B

Slowly raise your hands toward your forehead. When the incisional area starts to pull slightly, STOP AND HOLD THAT POSITION. Breathe deeply until the pulling stops. Continue raising your hands until you are able to reach the top of your head.

C If you have no incisional pain, slip your clasped hands down behind your neck. Keep your head erect.

In this exercise you should maintain your most advanced position as long as you can. When you tire, reverse the steps until your hands are back in your lap. It may take several sessions for you to accomplish the complete exercise but it may help to ease tensions in your neck and shoulder as well as make it easier for you to reach neck zippers and fix your hair.

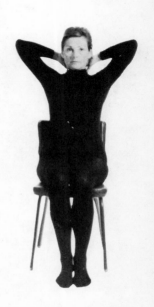

D Gradually spread your elbows apart remembering to stop and breathe deeply when pulling or pain occurs.

PULLEY

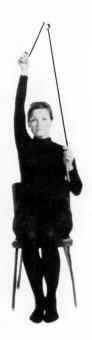

Please note special instructions if you have had a bilateral mastectomy.

Place the rope over a secure hook such as a clothes hook. Put a back of a chair under the rope.

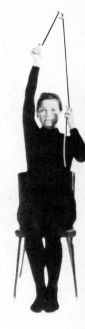

A

Sit up straight and grasp the rope as high as you can with your unaffected hand.

BILATERALS: Creep up the rope first with the fingers of the least painful arm. Stop when you feel incisional pain. Loop the rope around your fingers and keep your hand at that level.

B

With your affected arm, begin to reach or creep up the rope until you start to feel pain. Stop and loop the rope around your hand.

BILATERALS: Repeat A with the other hand.

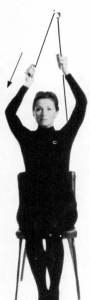

C

Pull your affected arm upward slowly by pulling down with your other arm. Stop when it hurts. Breathe deeply until the pain stops and repeat this part of the exercise. Eventually you will be able to get as high with the affected arm as with the unaffected.

BILATERALS: Let both arms hang limply in that position and breathe deeply until you have no incisional pulling or pain.

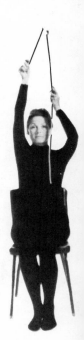

D

When you tire, unloop and slide slowly down with both hands at the same time.

BILATERALS: When you are comfortable, gently pull down on one side of the rope to raise the opposite arm. Stop when it hurts and breathe deeply. Then repeat this exercise using the opposite arm. When you have finished with both arms, slide both hands down the rope slowly.

Care of the Hand and Arm After Mastectomy

Swelling of the arm is seen in approximately 25 percent of women who have had thorough (radical) mastectomy, but in only 10 percent is the edema, or swelling, sufficiently marked so as to be handicapping.

A certain amount of swelling of the arm is seen immediately postoperatively in the majority of mastectomized patients but it tends to disappear within one to two weeks. If it persists beyond that time, the swelling is usually permanent.

Edema is seldom obvious if the circumference of the upper arm is increased less than two inches, or the forearm less than one inch. Of course, if the patient is very thin, a relatively smaller amount of edema may cause the arm to appear markedly swollen. Fortunately, people do not make it a habit to go around comparing the disparate sizes of their arms. If they did, they would note that a great many have one arm larger than the other. Manual workers such as carpenters, miners, and so on, who use one arm much more than the other during the course of their work, often have marked disparity in their two limbs.

Many attempts have been made to devise a satisfactory operation to overcome this lymphedema of the arm following mastectomy, but, to date, no successful procedure has been developed. Physical therapists, too, have concentrated on special exercises and treatments to relieve troublesome swelling, but they, too, have failed to come up with effective techniques. The best that can be done is to advise patients to try to sleep or rest with the arm on a pillow over one's head. Thus gravity will help drain the lymph, collected through the loss of lymph nodes and channels, out of the arm. Unfortunately, the maneuver is not always successful, as patients find it difficult to change from their usual resting or sleeping positions.

Women with exceptionally marked swelling of the arm frequently get some relief by wearing a specially designed elastic arm covering, much like an elastic stocking to support the leg. Others bandage their arms with elastic bandages, obtaining some relief. Both devices should be applied upon arising early in the morning before swelling has reached its maximum.

Because of the stagnation of lymph and the decreased number of antibodies and bacteria-fighting white blood cells occasioned by removal of the lymph nodes in the armpit, there is decreased resistance to infection in the involved arm. Estimates are that 8 to 10 percent of women who have had mastectomy will sooner or later develop an infection of the finger, hand, or arm. It is therefore important to observe several precautionary measures. These are:

1. Do not cut the fingernails too short in the corners. It may lead to a runaround (paronychia) infection. Also, do not file them too short in the corners.

2. Do not cut the cuticles with scissors. Instead, use a cuticle cream. A nick of the cuticle can lead to a paronychia infection.

3. Avoid the use of steel wool. If it must be used, wear heavy rubber gloves.

4. Be particularly careful with safety pins; avoid the small ones as they are more difficult to handle. Pinpricks can lead to finger infections.

5. Wear a thimble when sewing.

6. Do not scrub dishes, floors, or do any heavy cleaning with bare hands. Disposable plastic gloves are cheap and give good protection.

7. Wear heavy protective gloves when gardening. Avoid plants with thorns.

8. Wash thoroughly with mild soap and water any scratch or cut on the fingers or hands. Do not pour an antiseptic onto the area; it will do more harm than good.

9. Avoid detergents that might cause chapping of the hands. Infection can easily gain entrance through the cracks in the skin of chapped hands.

10. In cold weather, use hand lotions frequently.

11. Do not let your doctor vaccinate you on the involved arm.

12. Do not take injections, even antibiotics, in the involved arm.

13. Burns often become infected no matter where they occur; they are much more likely to become infected if they involve the arm on the side of a mastectomy. Therefore:

a. Hold your cigarette in the uninvolved hand.

b. Reach into the oven with the uninvolved hand.

c. Take hot things off the stove with the uninvolved hand.

d. Do not permit yourself to become too sunburned. Remember, sunburn is a real burn, in every sense.

14. Get into the habit of carrying heavy things with the uninvolved hand.

15. Avoid all constrictions about the finger, wrist, or arm, except an elastic device or bandage prescribed especially for you. Particularly:

a. Do not wear a short-sleeve blouse with elastic about the arms.

b. Do not wear rings that fit snugly.

c. Do not wear a snug-fitting bracelet or wristwatch.

d. Wear loose-fitting sleeves on your dresses.

16. *Never* use a hot water bag or electric pad on the affected arm.

Any infection on the affected side should prompt a visit to the physician. In all likelihood he will prescribe rest of the arm in an elevated position, warm moist soaks, a liberal fluid intake, and an antibiotic medication. Under this regime, the infection will subside within a few days.

A condition known as *lymphangitis* not infrequently develops in the affected arm. It can be diagnosed by tender, reddish streaks that may extend anywhere along the forearm or upper arm. The condition is caused by an inflammation of the lymph channels, possibly secondary to infection within a small scratch or cut in the hand. It is treated in the same manner as other infections described above. There should be no fear that these streaks represent a recurrence of the breast tumor.

Questions and Answers

Is it necessary for a woman who has had minor breast surgery to do exercises?

No.

Should all patients who have undergone mastectomy do exercises?

Yes. They are essential to full recovery.

Are postmastectomy exercises painful?
Not usually, unless one overreaches and strains too much.

Should cobalt, X-ray therapy, or chemotherapy interfere with the performance of the exercises?
No, even though it may be very tiring to continue them while undergoing therapy.

How does one contact the Reach to Recovery organization?
Call your local American Cancer Society office.

Is the arm on the side of a mastectomy much weaker than the arm on the unaffected side?
No, but the shoulder may tire more readily because of the absence of the pectoral muscles.

Is full use of the shoulder and arm usually restored after mastectomy?
Full use, or near full use.

Do all symptoms of mastectomy eventually subside?
Usually, but not always. Some women continue to have aching pain, numbness, and tingling sensations in the chest, shoulder, and arm for many years after mastectomy.

Why do some women get edema and others do not?
The cause is not known. Some investigators have felt that infection following mastectomy is conducive to edema, but this theory has not gained general acceptance. All agree that the basic cause is the removal of the lymph nodes and the interruption of the lymph channels in the armpit. However, the same dissection is carried out on those who don't get edema as those who do.

Are women who have had cobalt or high voltage X-ray therapy more likely to develop edema of their arms?
Some surgeons believe so, but most radiologists claim that radiation therapy does not have anything to do with postoperative swelling of the arm.

Is edema of the arm always obvious?

No, especially since most women with noticeable edema wear long-sleeved dresses.

Does arm swelling tend to disappear with the passage of time?

It may, but usually, only to a limited extent.

30 PSYCHOLOGICAL RECOVERY FROM BREAST SURGERY

Despite the elation that women with a benign lesion feel upon awakening from surgery to discover that their breast has not been removed, many of them become upset and depressed. It may even last for several weeks.

However, depression following mastectomy is profound. Patients often try to camouflage it to please their husband and children, but the feelings are present nevertheless.

Much can be done by the surgeon before he operates on his patient to mitigate the emotional upset after breast surgery. First and foremost, he must explain all the possibilities that might come to pass. He must be honest. If he thinks the breast will have to be removed, he should state so beforehand. This will give his patient time to adjust to the possibility and will minimize the shock that she experiences postoperatively.

When I was engaged in first-echelon battle surgery during World War II and on too many occasions was forced to amputate a shattered or gangrenous limb, I along with many of my colleagues soon learned that the soldier was better able to bear up under the loss if he was forewarned of the possibility. Those whose limbs were amputated without prior knowledge were the ones who found it most difficult to maintain emotional control postoperatively. The same situation is encountered over and over again in breast surgery.

It should be made abundantly clear to the patient about to undergo surgery that she might be forced to lose her breast but that such a loss is far preferable to losing her life. As she thinks over this awesome possibility, she will somehow reach the conclusion that it is not as bad as losing her sight, her hearing, or a limb. She will also come to realize that she will at least have one breast. (Fortunately, few women require removal of both breasts.) She should also be told that her life need not be altered to a great degree by the loss of her breast. Her sex life will remain the same; she will have full use of her arm on the involved side; no one need know that she has lost a breast, as it is simple to disguise the fact; she will be able to drive a car, to exercise, to swim and play golf or tennis; she will be able to resume all her household duties or return to her job.

Adjustments to reality crises are borne well by the integrated, productive individual. Women who break down after mastectomy are more often those who react poorly to all stressful situations. In other words, the neurotic woman is apt to react more severely to the loss of a breast. She must be treated with special kindness and understanding in order to avoid a serious, prolonged postoperative reaction. In my own practice I have never had a postoperative mastectomy patient who developed a postoperative psychosis. This fact is all the more interesting because postoperative psychosis is a complication of certain other types of major surgery, such as, occasionally, after a hysterectomy.

Patients who have undergone mastectomy must recover at their own pace. Relatives and friends who try to make believe nothing has transpired, and who ignore the patient's depressed mood, are not helping her toward recovery. If the patient wishes to discuss her situation with her family or friends, they should be willing to listen and should not change the subject. Postoperative mastectomy patients have a need to let go, to talk, to cry, to grieve. They should be encouraged to express themselves. After all, it is nonsensical to pretend that their experience was one of minor significance. The husband can play a vital role in helping his wife to reestablish stability by letting her know she still is physically attractive to him. One of my mastectomy patients told me the following story: The night she came home from the hospital her husband practically ripped off her clothes, threw her down on the bed, and began to make love to her. He spent considerable time caressing and kissing her normal breast, being careful not to touch the mastectomy wound area that was covered with dressings. She was thrilled by his ardor and unexpectedly found herself responding in kind. She began to cry after the lovemaking reached its climax, but, she said, they were tears of joy.

This patient has never gone through any real postoperative depression, and she attributes it to the fact that her husband never let her feel she was in any way different to him.

Time is nature's greatest healer, and women who have undergone mastectomy eventually adjust to their special problem and become increasingly more cheerful as time goes on. Within a few months after their operation they begin to resume their role in their family, among their friends, and in business. Many of them develop great pride in surmounting their tribulations and become actively engaged in helping others toward recovery.

The organization Reach to Recovery has done remarkably good work in helping mastectomy patients to physical as well as psychological recovery. They send women who have themselves recovered from breast cancer to visit recently operated patients while they are still in the hospital. It is a great comfort for those who have just undergone this type of surgery to have contact with women who are fully recovered, cheerful, and living full lives many years after their mastectomy. It is then that they begin to realize they, too, can surmount the trauma of their operation.

The long-term care of those who have undergone breast removal is sometimes hampered by the patients' conscious or unconscious desire to shut the memory of the painful experience completely out of their minds. As a result, they ignore their doctor's admonitions to return for periodic checkups. Instead of coming in every 4 or 6 months, they not infrequently permit much longer periods to elapse between examinations. When confronted with the fact that they have been remiss in their duty toward themselves, these women usually respond with complete frankness that they thought their previous checkup had been much more recent. Since regular reexamination of the operative site *and* the opposite breast is essential to good long-term care, the patients must be lectured sternly if they get into the habit of neglecting their visits. Those who fail to return regularly should be sent a reminder card when their periodic examination becomes due.

Questions and Answers

Should the woman who has undergone mastectomy be encouraged to return to normal living as soon as she is physically able to do so?

Yes, within limits. A markedly depressed woman *cannot* be forced into normal living. Such attempts may stimulate strong negative responses.

How long does a patient's depressed state usually last after breast surgery?

Anywhere from a few weeks to several months. The more stable a woman was before surgery, the more quickly will she recover.

Are there any medications to relieve depressed feelings after breast surgery?

Yes. There are tranquilizers and medications that can be given to overcome a depressed state. However, they are not always helpful inasmuch as the depressed state is due to a reality situation, not a fantasy one. A doctor should always be consulted before taking any of these drugs.

Can consultation with a psychiatrist help the depressed postoperative patient?

Yes, if the depression is deep and unusually prolonged.

Do women eventually recover from the emotional upset caused by breast removal?

Yes. Time factors vary, but recovery eventually takes place.

31 THE MALE BREAST

Studies of plant and animal life over the eons indicate that Nature has always been a great experimenter, taking all sorts of biological risks in creating life forms that lasted a relatively short time and had little chance for ultimate survival. Thus, we note huge numbers of plants and animals that have become extinct millions of years ago, and an ever-growing number that are becoming extinct today.

And even when we inspect Homo sapiens, alleged to be Nature's most illustrious accomplishment, it is obvious that the job could have been done much better! As an example, let us consider the male breast, a structure encountered in all mammals. What did Nature have in mind for this decorative appendage? Was it supposed to serve a real purpose, or was it a whimsical act committed during a moment when Nature was in a joking mood?

The male breast is a difficult thing to understand in the light of our knowledge that the sex of a mammal is decided at the very instant an egg is fertilized by a sperm. The female egg, that is, the ovum, and the male sperm each have 23 chromosomes; 22 of the chromosomes in the ovum are just like 22 of the chromosomes found in the male sperm. However, the female egg always has an X-sex chromosome as its 23rd chromosome, whereas only half the male sperm have an X-sex chromosome; the other half are Y. If the egg is fertilized by a sperm containing an X-sex chromosome, the developing embryo will become a girl. If the egg is fertilized by a sperm containing a Y-sex chromosome, a boy will eventuate. Thus, at the instant of fertilization, sex is determined, yet for several weeks thereafter, the embryo continues to form cells that could serve either sex. Indeed, a strange happening.

Anatomically, the breast of a newborn male is identical to that of the newborn female. And, as mentioned elsewhere in this book, both the male and female breast sometimes produce milk for a few days after the child is born. This phenomenon results from the female hormone secretions of the mother that have been passed through the placenta and into the circulation of the unborn infant. As the male child grows, his breast remains a relatively rudimentary structure and any secreting gland tissue that was present at birth becomes inactive. Male breast tissue consists mainly of ducts and intervening blood vessels.

On the role of the male breast as a sex organ, the literature contains very little information. In fact, it seldom plays an active role, although a certain amount of pleasure is felt when the female presses her breasts against the male's. Men display little reaction if their mates manipulate or kiss their nipples, and this type of stimulation alone seldom evokes an erection. Of course, there are exceptions to every generality, and when discussing sex, the number of variations from standard practice is enormous. I had a patient who could attain an erection only when he manipulated his own nipples; and a colleague's patient insisted that his wife anoint her nipples with cold cream and then rub them against his nipples. The patient was unable to initiate intercourse without this strange maneuver.

The male breast therefore has no known function and is not subject to the same cyclic influences that affect the female breast from the pre-adolescent years through the menopause. However, certain changes do occur in the male breast as the result of increased amounts of male hormone circulating in the bloodstream prior to and during adolescence—and then again in the later years when the amount of male hormone diminishes. These changes will be discussed later in this chapter, as will the influence of the female hormone on the male breast.

Almost all the birth deformities that are seen in the female breast may also occur in the male breast. As a matter of fact, supernumerary or extra nipples are seen somewhat more often in the male than in the female. However, supernumerary nipples in the male are rarely accompanied by any underlying breast tissue. Consequently, when adolescence takes place, there is no increase in the size of the nipples. No treatment is necessary for this anomaly, but if the nipple is large or if it causes self-consciousness, it is a simple matter to excise it surgically. Amastia, or absence of a breast, can also occur in the male but, naturally, the anomaly has much less significance than when encountered in a female.

As one might expect from the fact that the male breast is a functionless structure, it is seldom influenced by the ordinary changes that take place in body function. Despite this, the male breast either is occasionally the primary site of a disease process or is affected by a systemic disorder. The main conditions affecting the male breast are:

1. Milk secretion, already mentioned, caused by the female hormones transmitted to the unborn infant by its mother. If one of the major milk ducts is obstructed and the milk dams up behind the obstruction, the stagnant fluid may become secondarily infected, and the infant develops a breast abscess, requiring incision and drainage. Quick recovery is the general rule.

2. An adolescent nodule, that small, round, firm swelling beneath the nipple seen occasionally in boys between the ages of 11 and 15 years. It may involve one or both nipples. Occasionally, one nodule will disappear, and a short time later the other nipple develops a similar nodule. The adolescent nodule is thought to be associated with the increased secretion of male sex hormone (androgen) that takes place just prior to the onset of puberty.

A considerable amount of tenderness may be experienced with this condition when the nipple is touched or when the child lies upon it in bed.

The adolescent nodule requires no treatment, and will disappear spontaneously within a few months to a year's time. The boy and his parents must be assured that the lump does *not* represent tumor formation and that biopsy is unnecessary.

3. Gynecomastia is by far the most common disorder affecting the male breast. The term *gynecomastia* means "female breast," and is characterized by breast enlargement. On microscopic examination of a breast involved in gynecomastia, one finds true glandular tissue. This type of tissue is absent or present only in minute quantities in the normal male breast.

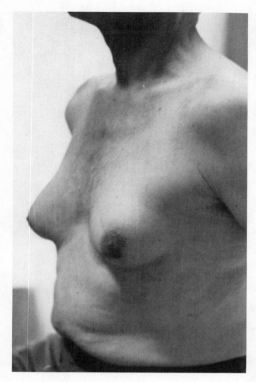

Gynecomastia in a man receiving estrogen in the treatment of a malignancy of the prostate gland.

Nipple one year after subcutaneous removal of a male breast involved in gynecomastia.

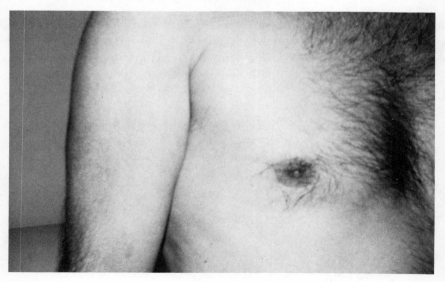

Most cases of gynecomastia are of unknown origin and are not associated with systemic disease or with a disorder in glandular metabolism (endocrine function). It is frequently seen in young men in their twenties or thirties who are just as virile and masculine as their less protuberant friends. However, the condition does cause a great deal of embarrassment, especially when the person becomes the target of jibes and jokes about his "femininity." Gynecomastia more often affects both breasts, but it may occur on one side only.

Gynecomastia of unknown origin is very common in older men in their fifties, sixties, or seventies, and is more often one-sided, although it may involve both breasts, too. Unilateral gynecomastia may create a good deal of anxiety, especially in older men, because of the fear that the swelling is due to cancer.

Although most cases of gynecomastia fall into the *idiopathic* (unknown origin) category, there are some cases associated with abnormal physiological states or with disease processes elsewhere in the body. It might be well to enumerate these conditions:

a. Adolescent gynecomastia. This type of breast enlargement is thought to result from an increase in the amount of male sex hormone circulating in the blood. Its onset is during early puberty and it tends to subside as adolescence proceeds toward maturity.

b. Gynecomastia is encountered frequently among boys who have *undescended testicles.* This type is thought to be the result of inadequate amounts of male sex hormone in the circulating blood.

c. Gynecomastia is occasionally noted among boys with birth defects such as hypospadias (an abnormal opening of the urethra in the penis) or with Klinefelter's syndrome, a congenital condition in which the testicles are underdeveloped and are unable to produce sperm.

d. Gynecomastia may be seen in patients with cancer of the adrenal gland, tumors of the testicle, cirrhosis of the liver, hepatitis, liver tumor, or overactivity of the thyroid gland.

e. Gynecomastia secondary to prolonged starvation was seen in more than 10 percent of men who spent long periods in Nazi concentration camps during World War II.

f. Strange as it seems, gynecomastia can be produced by giving a man either the male or female sex hormone in large quantities.

Aging men do take male sex hormone in order to maintain their waning potency. Others, because of an injury or disease of the testicles, may require male hormone to enable them to copulate. In either event, a by-product of this therapy may be breast enlargement.

It is common practice for men with cancer of the prostate gland to be given large doses of female sex hormone (estrogen) to slow the growth of the tumor. Some urologists believe that this form of treatment can keep a patient with prostatic cancer alive for many extra years. In almost all cases where this treatment is given, the male breast will grow to such proportions that it resembles the female organ. For this reason, urologists may recommend removal of all breast tissue beneath the nipple prior to instituting estrogen therapy.

g. Gynecomastia secondary to drugs is not infrequently encountered. It may follow the prolonged use of digitalis, diuretics, drugs to reduce high blood pressure, amphetamines, or other medications. Within a few weeks after the drug has been discontinued, the breast returns to normal or near-normal size.

h. Pseudogynecomastia is a condition in which the breast appears to be enlarged but, in actuality, the enlargement is due solely to obesity. The breast subsides when normal weight is regained.

Although surgical treatment for gynecomastia in young men is usually not essential, it is often requested for cosmetic or psychological reasons. Young men in the armed forces often seek removal of their enlarged breasts to avoid the embarrassment it creates. When such relief is sought, it should be granted.

Gynecomastia of unknown origin in older men should be treated surgically in order to be absolutely certain that cancer is not present.

The surgical treatment for gynecomastia consists of removing all the breast tissue that lies beneath and adjacent to the nipple. The nipple need not be removed in performing this operation. A semicircular incision is made in the outer perimeter of the nipple, the nipple is reflected and all the underlying tissue is removed. The reflected portion of the nipple is then replaced and is stitched back to its surrounding skin. This operation is *subcutaneous mastectomy,* performed under light general anesthesia. The patient is confined to the hospital for two to three days. In cases with unusually large breasts, the operative procedure requires more dissection and more time to carry out. Also, because of oozing from the deeper tissues, it may be necessary to insert a rubber drain and to keep the patient in the hospital for a few extra days.

The wounds following subcutaneous mastectomy in the male heal within seven to ten days, leaving behind a minimal scar. Since all the breast tissue is removed, it cannot grow back again.

When performing surgery on an older man with gynecomastia, it is common practice to do a frozen-section biopsy of the excised tissue while the patient is still under anesthesia. In this way, absolute assurance can be given that no cancer is present.

4. Although the male breast can harbor a benign tumor such as a fibroadenoma or cyst, this condition is very rare. Most

benign lesions occur in the gland tissue of the breast and since the normal male breast has so little glandular structure, one would not expect to find disorders of glandular origin. On the other hand, the male breast does have ducts, and lesions of these structures are encountered once in a while. Intraductal papillomas, the warty growths found in the lining of the ducts, are rare in the male breast. (I have seen only two such cases in more than forty years of surgery.) An intraductal papilloma will evidence itself by a clear-colored, straw-colored, or bloody discharge from the nipple. In most cases, a frank tumor will not be felt beneath the nipple.

Any discharge from the male breast (in an individual not receiving hormones) should be an indication for a biopsy. Although intraductal papillomas are almost always benign, they can develop into cancer and their early removal may prevent such an eventuality. The preferred procedure in these cases is subcutaneous mastectomy, the same operation as in gynecomastia.

5. Cancer of the male breast occurs one hundred times less frequently than in the female. When it affects the male, he is usually in his late fifties, sixties, or seventies.

The diagnosis of breast cancer in the male, unfortunately, often is made much later on in the course of the disease than in the female. This can be attributed to the fact that men do not think of themselves as candidates for this disease and they therefore tend to neglect warning signs. Physicians, too, contribute to late diagnosis as many omit routine breast examination in the male. As a result of late diagnosis, the outlook for survival or cure of male breast cancer is lower than that in the female.

Signs that should alert a man to seek breast examination include the finding of a lump—no matter how small—underneath the nipple, a discharge from the nipple, retraction of the nipple, any crusting or ulceration of the nipple that fails to heal within a week or two.

The treatment for cancer of the male breast is the same

as that for female breast cancer. In the majority of cases, if the malignancy is still confined to the breast and to the lymph nodes (glands) in the armpit, a thorough (radical) mastectomy is indicated. If the lymph nodes are found to be involved, cobalt therapy and/or chemotherapy are indicated. See chapter titled "Breast Cancer."

Questions and Answers

Do males ever get breast infections?
Yes, but not nearly as often as females. Syphilis and tuberculosis have been known to attack the male breast.

Is a lump in a male breast ever caused by an inflammation?
Yes, a male breast can develop an abscess, or it may become inflamed by an infection such as tuberculosis, syphilis, or any other bacterial invader.

Do males have breast birth deformities?
Yes, similar to those in the female.

Do adolescent nodules ever develop into gynecomastia?
Some boys who have had an adolescent nodule may later develop gynecomastia, but often no cause-and-effect relationship exists between the two conditions.

Do adolescent boys ever get enlargement of both breasts?
Yes. The secretion of a substance similar to the female sex hormone may be circulating in a preadolescent boy's blood. As the testicles mature, the male sex hormone is secreted in larger quantities and the breasts stop enlarging. As adolescents reach maturity, the breasts appear smaller.

Can an adolescent boy retain enlarged breasts even when he has matured?
Yes.

Is there a tendency for gynecomastia to be inherited?
Yes. It will often be found that the father had the same condition.

Do men who have enlarged breasts tend to be less fertile than those who do not?

No. It has been found that the sex development of the male, including his fertility and potency, have nothing whatever to do with gynecomastia.

Is gynecomastia painful?
No.

Are operations for gynecomastia successful?
Yes, invariably.

Do breasts ever grow back again after surgery?
No, since the operation for gynecomastia consists of removing all the breast tissue beneath the nipple.

Is there much of a scar left following excision of the male breast?
No, unless the gynecomastia is very large. In such cases, the semicircular incision may be extended in a medial and lateral direction for an inch or two. This will leave a visible scar.

Is the nipple ever deformed after an operation for gynecomastia?
This occurs sometimes, but the deformity is not great.

Should hormone treatment be given to men who have enlarged breasts?
No. There is no satisfactory hormone treatment for gynecomastia.

If gynecomastia exists secondary to a disease in another organ, will it subside when the primary disease is brought under control?
In some cases; in others, the gynecomastia will persist despite the fact that the related disease has been arrested. Consideration should then be given to surgical excision of the enlarged breast.

Is gynecomastia ever associated with tenderness of the breast?
Yes, in some instances, especially in those in the older age groups.

Do aging men ever develop pendulous breasts?

Yes. This is not true gynecomastia, but merely the sagging of enlarged breasts.

Can plastic surgery help men with gynecomastia?

Yes, if the man is vain enough to want corrective surgery, it is completely feasible.

Are operations for plastic repair of the male breast successful?

Yes.

Are men who are on prolonged administration of female sex hormones more likely to develop cancer of their breasts?

Yes. It has been found that such patients occasionally will develop cancer.

Is gynecomastia ever secondary to the administration of the male sex hormone?

Yes. Many men who take male sex hormone to increase their potency will, after a period of several weeks or months, develop enlargement of their breasts.

Will gynecomastia tend to disappear after the cessation of the female or male sex hormones?

Yes, the breasts will tend to return to normal, but they may not do so completely.

Is enlargement of the male breast in older men usually associated with loss of virility?

No. Enlargement of the male breast is no gauge of the virility or potency of a man.

Does idiopathic gynecomastia affecting both breasts tend to disappear by itself?

No. This condition tends to persist indefinitely.

How can a doctor distinguish between benign gynecomastia and a cancer of the breast?

Gynecomastia usually involves all the breast tissue beneath the nipple.

It will therefore form a rubbery, rounded, circular area involving all the tissue beneath the nipple. A cancer of the breast feels irregular, very hard, and usually does not involve all the tissue beneath the nipple. In addition, cancer of the male breast is sometimes associated with a discharge or ulceration of the nipple, and enlargement of the glands in the armpit.

Are operations on the male breast dangerous?
No. Even radical surgery for cancer can be tolerated if the patient is in satisfactory general health.

Will a male respond to chemical therapy as satisfactorily as a female following cancer of the breast?
Yes.

Is removal of the testicles ever indicated in treating a cancer of the male breast that has spread to other organs?
No. The continued production of male sex hormone does not seem to influence the growth of breast cancer in the male.

Does the nipple of the male breast contain nerve endings that produce erotic sensations?
It is curious that microscopic examination of the male nipple is practically a duplication of that seen in the female. In other words, the same nerve endings are present in the male and female, yet the male rarely feels sexual stimulation by having his nipples manipulated or kissed.

INDEX